Vitamin B₆
The Doctor's Report

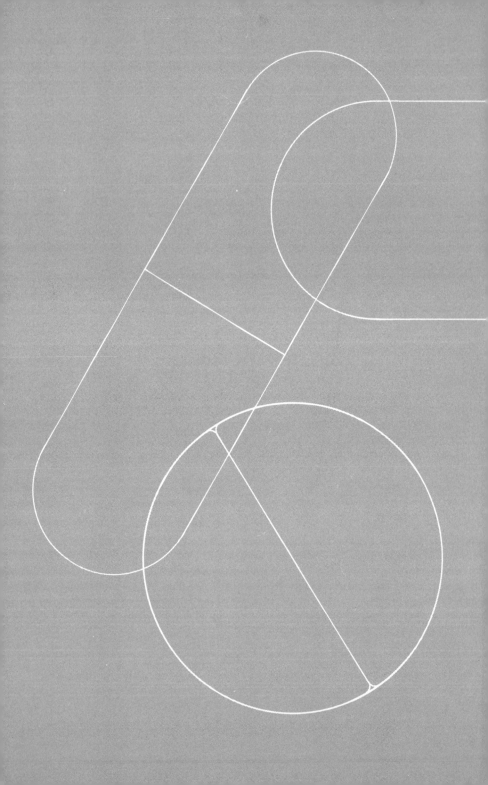

Vitamin B$_6$
The Doctor's Report

John M. Ellis, M.D. &
James Presley

1817

Harper & Row, Publishers
New York, Evanston, San Francisco, London

FIRST EDITION

Designed by Patricia Dunbar

Library of Congress Cataloging in Publication Data

Ellis, John M
    Vitamin B₆: the doctor's report.
    Bibliography: p.
    1. Pyridoxine deficiency.   2. Vitamin therapy.
I. Presley, James, joint author.   II. Title.
[DNLM: 1. Pyridoxine.   2. Pyridoxine deficiency.
QU 195 E47v 1973]
RC620.5.E53   615'.328   72-9753
ISBN 0-06-011171-2

For

our

wives, Lucille Ellis and Fran Presley,

with love

Editor's Note

Although vitamin B_6 has been proven to be a nontoxic vitamin, it is suggested that the reader first check with his own physician before making an assumption as to what the prescribed daily requirement should be.

Contents

Preface

It is a great scientific satisfaction and pleasure to write a note as preface to the book *Vitamin B₆: The Doctor's Report.*

The authors have succeeded in bringing to light not only the history of vitamin B₆ but also more recent developments leading to the clinical-metabolic role of the vitamin.

The late 1920s represented the heroic age of vitamin research, in particular the complicated analysis of the vitamin B complex. I was active with my associates in identifying in the B complex, in addition to the long-known beriberi factor (B_1), three new vitamins: riboflavin, B_6 (pyridoxine), and biotin. An unexpected special premium of this study was recognition of these new vitamins—starting with riboflavin—as co-enzymes in a large number of enzymes, thus basically as pro-enzymes. Credit is due to E. E. Snell[1] * and his associates for first recognizing the existence of other forms of pyridoxine—i.e., pyridoxal and pyridoxamine. Pyridoxine, pyridoxamine, and pyridoxal owe their B_6 activity to the ability of the organism to convert them through enzymatic pathways to the co-enzyme form, pyridoxal-5-phosphate. To quote A. E. Braunstein, the famous Soviet biochemist: "Pyridoxal phosphate holds an exceptional place among the co-enzymes with regard both to the unparalleled diversity of its catalytic function and to their paramount significance in biochemical transformations of amino acids and in integral pattern of nitrogen metabolism."[2] A recent tabulation listed over fifty pyridoxal-phosphate-dependent enzymes and the corresponding catalyzed reactions.[3]

With this cellular-biochemical background, it could not be considered a surprise that in the last twenty years the number of clinical-pathological manifestations of direct or indirect vitamin B_6 deficiency increased in rapid succession.

The book of Ellis and Presley brings a complete, detached and, where necessary, critical new summary of all these B_6-linked syndromes and symptoms. In particular, emphasis should be placed on the completely new observations put forth by the untiring, often intuitive, efforts of the authors, especially those of John M. Ellis, who became a true pioneer for the assessment of vitamin B_6 metabolic disturbances. His clinical results with high pyridoxine doses in edematous conditions, in forms of rheumatism, "carpal tunnel" syndrome, menopausal arthritis, various clinical disturbances after the use of antiovulatory pills and many others, require thorough reading of his book. *Vitamin B_6: The Doctor's Report* is a true success story.

Paul György, M.D., M.D.h.c.

* Source notes begin on page 233.

Vitamin B_6
The Doctor's Report

Tingling Fingers, Cramps, and "Dead" Hands | I

The two patients, man and wife, came to me that day* with, literally, a double handful of troubles.

"Doctor," said the husband, a slender, wiry man of fifty-two, "my hands feel like pins and needles are sticking in them. They're painful and they hurt, and now I've lost my job because I can't use them.

"I can't use a razor to shave off my whiskers! For the last several weeks my daughter has had to shave me. I can't even grip the handle of a skillet with enough strength to pick it up. It takes both hands to hold the handle.

"And I've had to get someone to drive for me. My fingers would cramp and coil and lock around the steering wheel, and I would have to get somebody to pull 'em apart for me."

His nights were as agonizing as his days. Almost every night he was forced from his bed in violent pain because of "charlie horses," as he called the nocturnal muscle spasms and cramps in his legs. Several times he had struck matches to apply heat to the knotted muscles in his legs. Nothing had helped. Each night he lost several hours of sleep, and when morning came he wasn't any better off.

* February 11, 1969.

He had to roll out of bed awkwardly, like an invalid old man, on his hands and knees.

And, as if these were not afflictions enough for one man, he complained bitterly of pain in his arms, shoulders, and chest.

My patient D. J.'s condition had forced him into early retirement because his livelihood depended particularly on his manual dexterity. He had worked in a poultry-processing plant that had a volume of several thousand chickens daily. With his hands and fingers moving constantly, his job was to remove the intestines and viscera of the fowls as they passed before him on a mechanical conveyor belt. Over a period of many weeks his hands had become progressively crippled. One day he could no longer perform the job he had been hired to do. He lost his job, and his employer lost a hard-working, reliable employee.

In his medical history he had had no serious illness, operation, or injury. As I carefully examined him physically, I could find no abnormalities, except for the extremities of which he complained. He pointed to an area over his heart where he had felt the chest pains, but my findings were negative. As I listened through my stethoscope, his heart sounds were strong, with the volume and tone good.

His hands were another matter. There I found a network of medical problems, as if everything wrong with him had consolidated and coalesced in his hands. He couldn't flex his fingers at the middle, or interphalangeal, joints. When he tried to flex his fingers rapidly, involuntary muscle spasms shot up his forearms, and the severe pain in the finger joints made him shift in his chair. Even my touching his finger joints with relatively little pressure brought discomfort. Furthermore, his fingertips had lost their delicate touch sensation, the ability to distinguish between wood or paper or cloth.

Inspecting his hands closely, I perceived a slight swelling, or edema, of the fingers and hands. Then I touched the skin of his palm. His hands were cold and clammy and perspiring slightly.

Surprisingly, in view of the other features of his crippled hands, he could still make a kind of fist, and his metacarpophalangeal joints—those joints where the fingers join the hand, which we call the knuckles—functioned and were free of pain.

His wife, H. J., forty-three, had problems almost as serious, although she hadn't lost her job yet. She had begun to drop objects, such as a skillet while in the kitchen, and to break dishes where she worked. During the past five months she had been a dishwasher at two different well-known restaurants in the area.

The dropping of objects had gradually come to be for her a serious sign of disease, and, like her husband, she had tingling hands combined with a numbness that made them "feel like they are dead." The tingling felt "just like needles are sticking in my fingers and hands."

Her left shoulder was so filled with pain that she couldn't raise her arm over her head high enough to comb her hair. One knee joint was so painfully swollen that she couldn't flex the knee while sitting.

In another city she had received an injection, presumably hydrocortisone, in the knee joint twice a month for seven months. The injection had reduced the pain and swelling for a few days; then it had relentlessly returned. She had also taken a pain pill daily, along with another pill for nausea, and lately she had been taking about eight aspirins a day. The aspirins eased the pain to some extent but had no effect on the swelling. By the time she came to my office the knee had gone untreated for several weeks.

"I can't ride in the back seat of a car with my leg drawn up at the knee," she said. "I have to hold my leg straight. I can't bend my knee that much."

An examination confirmed all this. She grimaced each time she attempted to raise her left arm at the shoulder. Her hands and fingers were swollen. The middle joints of her fingers would not flex completely and easily. Her left knee, appearing obese, was swollen. It was stiff. She cried out when I tried to flex her knee for her.

The symptoms (subjective evidence, reported by the patient) and signs (objective evidence, apparent to me and others) of disease conditions that D. J. and H. J. presented were hardly new to me by then, although D. J. seemed to have more of the classical symptoms than I usually found in one person. These included tingling fingers, nocturnal muscle spasms and cramps or "charlie horses" in the legs, numbness in the hands as if they were dead, painful locking of the finger joints (trigger finger), severe pains in the arms, shoulders, and chest, and edema, or swelling. In my thirty years of medical experience that included twenty years of private practice, I had examined thousands of patients with similar symptoms, from all walks of life and socio-economic classes, young and old, white and black, rich and poor. During ten of those years I had had extensive experience with an unusual, but uncomplicated, therapy. With this clinical knowledge, I prescribed for D. J. and H. J. the same simple medication with which I had treated thousands of other patients: vitamin B_6 in the form of pyridoxine tablets.

I instructed both D. J. and H. J. to take a 50-milligram tablet of pyridoxine twice a day, morning and night—a daily total for each of 100 milligrams of vitamin B_6. At this point I made no effort to modify their diets. No drug, no other medication was prescribed. The B_6 tablets constituted the only change whatsoever.

When they returned to my office three weeks later, the patients themselves told the story as well as anybody could.

"Last Sunday before last," said D. J., "I shaved myself for the first time [in months]. On the fifth morning after I started taking the medicine [i.e., vitamin B_6], I could shave myself with a straight razor. My daughter didn't have to shave me.

"I don't have that ol' tingling and aching in my hands. Most of my fingers I can move and they will not swell, but if I move this one"—he pointed to the proximal interphalangeal joint of the long finger of one hand—"several times, it swells."

Now he could drive his automobile, whereas previously he had had to find someone to drive for him. His cramps had virtually subsided. He could get out of bed as a normal person did. The tingling and numbness—"it'd feel kinda like your hand would go to sleep"—were gone. He had a firmer hand grip, and his palms were no longer cold and sweaty. Now, for instance, he could squeeze water out of a rag, which he had been unable to do before taking B_6 for three weeks.

He said that he still experienced what he described as "vibrations" in his hands—apparently residual tingling.

As I ran him through a series of motor tests, I found an improvement in range and speed of finger flexion and reduced finger pain from movement and pressure. The diffuse swelling in his fingers and hands had subsided, along with spasms in the forearm muscles when I had him flex his fingers rapidly. His hands were warm and dry. Tactile sensation in his fingertips had improved, and his hand grip was obviously stronger.

The relief that vitamin B_6 had brought D. J.'s wife was just as dramatic.

"I couldn't draw my knee up three weeks ago," H. J. said. "I couldn't straighten it or bend it. Now I can ride in the back seat of a car with my leg drawn up at the knee. There is a whole lot of difference in the swelling. I can wear a garter now. Then I couldn't."

Now she could raise her arms to comb her hair. This was the first time she had been free of pain in her shoulder and arm for a period of from seven to eight months. She had noticed a recession of symptoms, she said, within three to four days after starting the B_6 therapy.

Her hand grip was stronger. She could hold objects better. She could grasp a skillet firmly now. The numbness and tingling in her hands and fingers had subsided. She raised her arm above her head without suffering pain in the left shoulder. There was some residual, but less, pain in her knee joint, although the swelling had vanished. She demonstrated definitely improved finger flexion at the interphalangeal joints.

I told her to continue, indefinitely, to take 50 milligrams of pyridoxine a day and to resume her regular routine.

Three weeks later D. J. returned for his third office visit. His improvement continued to be exciting, as exhibited in improved finger flexion and reduced pain. Normal sensation had been restored to his fingers. His hands were still warm and dry and his hand grip was normal. He could hold his fingers in sustained flexion without muscle spasms or locking of the finger joints. His nocturnal muscle spasms were now definitely a thing of the past.

For this six-week period, from February 11 to March 25 of that year, he had been off his job, during which time his hands and fingers had had an extended respite from vigorous exercise. During the recovery period he noted that, at first, exercise made his finger joints more painful and more swollen, but after four weeks of treatment with vitamin B₆ he could exercise vigorously without suffering.

He continued to have chest pain, he concluded, but it was not as severe as it had been before treatment. I asked him if he had done any exercise during the past week. He replied that he had been working with a hoe and shovel while planting a home vegetable garden—a form of vigorous exercise.

The pessimism I had seen on his first visit had been supplanted by an aura of optimism and hope. Once again he had control of his hands. He could work now, and he wanted to. He intended to leave town, to look for another job, and, instructing him to take 50 milligrams of pyridoxine daily and indefinitely, I saw no medical reason why he shouldn't.

On his record I entered the same final diagnosis that I had written on his wife's chart: "Rheumatism—responsive to pyridoxine."

D. J. and H. J. had become a part of the growing body of scientific, clinical documentation of the vital medical powers of vitamin B₆, one of our most essential human nutrients—if one nutrient can be so described. These two patients had been stricken and crippled in what could have been the prime of life for both of them. They had been left physical wrecks and economic ciphers. Then, without drugs or regimentation of diet, they both had been restored to health and to use of their hands, at the cost of a few pennies a day. To that couple, who had just about given up on life, and their family, it must have seemed little short of miraculous.

Significantly, in these two case histories both D. J. and his wife H. J. complained of the same symptoms of numbness, tingling, and a "dead" sensation in their hands. These symptoms were a common affliction of many patients. Frequently there was a puffy swelling about the finger joints. Moving the fingers caused pain, particularly on waking in the morning. Wedding rings were tight and often were difficult to remove. For some, even the mildest of handshakes brought intense pain. Middle-aged women, in particular, seemed to have this trouble most, and these patients were also concerned about the exquisitely tender and reddened little bony knots that appeared on the sides of their finger joints. There was an air of resignation in most of the patients. They referred to their condition as "arthritis" and, shrugging their shoulders, accepted it with little hope of cure.

But by using, in succession, a balanced vitamin diet, a series of vitamin B-complex injections, a series of B_6 injections, and, finally, B_6 tablets only, I had learned that in most instances the patient could be restored to health. My first clinical proof of this vitamin's value came when I discovered, in working with patients in private practice, that numbness and tingling (paresthesia) and swelling (edema) would respond to B_6. From that point on I began using B_6 extensively in treating a number of disease conditions that had previously not been known to respond to B_6. Detailed histories were taken of patients who I suspected might benefit from the nutrient. Symptom by symptom, sign by sign, a relationship to B_6 was established. Objective before-and-after-treatment data were compiled through photographs and motion pictures.

In order to keep my patients' B_6 levels high, I repeatedly prescribed B_6 tablets, in the form of pyridoxine hydrochloride, usually stipulating 50 milligrams a day. Scores of patients have now taken B_6 for more than eight years, and thousands have done so for at least five years, all without ill effects. The principle of *Primum non nocere*—Latin for "Above all, do no harm"—is dutifully followed in B_6 therapy. B_6 is a water-soluble vitamin; any excess taken into the system is excreted in the urine within eight hours after ingestion. Unlike vitamins A and D, for instance, which are fat-soluble, it cannot store up in the liver. As it is with vitamin C and other B-complex vitamins, we must get a fresh supply each day. Therefore, vitamin B_6, unlike a drug, is a nutrient that can't harm the patient but very possibly can help him.

After a period of time it became evident that more than just "plain old rheumatism" was involved in the patients' complaints. The more I studied the pattern of symptoms and signs, the clearer it became that a wide sampling of the population was affected. These same symptoms related to disease conditions that hadn't been linked together in this way before. The symptoms and signs were spread among patients suffering from diabetes, heart disease, rheumatism, certain forms of arthritis, those taking birth-control pills, and those pregnant. All of these patients responded well to

B$_6$. If older patients were in the later stages of diabetes or heart disease, B$_6$ would not at that point reverse insulin requirements or prevent eventual myocardial infarction, since these were conditions that had been long years in the forming, but accompanying symptoms did respond to B$_6$.

In the course of the investigation the question arose: Was the disturbance of function in these cases primarily in the circulation of the blood, or was it in the *nerves* of the hands? In the seventeenth century an English physician, William Harvey, had discovered how blood circulates in the heart, arteries, and veins. His book *An Anatomical Treatise on the Motion of the Blood in Animals*, published in 1628, became a cornerstone in medicine. Since that time the scientific community has been working with great emphasis on the circulation and the circulatory system. However, when one thinks of a vitamin and the enzymatic reactions in which it is involved, one has to think of *all* systems in the body. Of these one thinks especially of the nervous system, because deficiencies of the B vitamins very quickly cause functional changes in the brain and the nerves that come from the spinal cord. Vitamin B$_6$, in playing its crucial role in human nutrition, is necessary for the metabolism of protein in millions of human body cells. It enters into more than fifty enzymatic reactions involving cells in the brain, liver, nerves, blood vessels, kidneys, muscles, and the ductless glands that produce certain hormones. For the body to function in normal health and to meet the stresses of ordinary modern living, all our food must be efficiently utilized. Without sufficient vitamin B$_6$ we cannot utilize our protein properly. Thus, its importance is without question.

It took years for me to conclude finally that a sustained need for B$_6$ was causing changes in the hands through ways other than disturbances in circulation. The changes primarily were in the nerves of the hand and in the function of the tendons that move the fingers. As the B$_6$ story unfolds, additional case histories will bring this out in detail. It was a fascinating revelation that, although B$_6$ might be changing the circulatory system, it is also definitely important in the function of two other systems: the nervous system and the musculoskeletal system.

For a number of reasons it now appears that vitamin B$_6$ may well be a link in the prevention of a number of diseases that have long been centers of medical controversy, such as rheumatism, diabetes, arteriosclerosis or hardening of the arteries, and associated heart attacks of the coronary occlusion type. Laboratory evidence has been mounting for several years to support this.

From early studies that involved crippled and tingling hands and swelling, the success of B_6 therapy finally spread to include at least eight disease conditions, which are to be discussed in this book. These are: latent edema, or swelling, in the hands, feet, and bodies of thousands of patients; the edema of pregnancy; premenstrual edema; edema and abdominal swelling associated with the use of the antiovulatory, or birth control, pills; rheumatism; the shoulder-hand syndrome; the carpal tunnel (wrist-hand) syndrome; and menopausal arthritis. Of these, at least six—the four conditions of edema plus menopausal arthritis and the carpal tunnel syndrome—involve the hormones. The shoulder-hand syndrome is intimately related to symptoms of heart disease. There is also a relationship, frequently, between some of these symptoms and diabetes.

One of the best indexes of disease has always been the deviation from the normal. A physician uses this daily as a means of diagnosis. The patient recognizes his symptoms by the same guide. But what is normal? Since in this book we will be dealing over and over with the hands, face, and feet, let us discuss these portions of the anatomy in order to establish what is normal.

First, let us look at the hand. The hand functions primarily for purposes of flexion, which is to say grasping and clutching things. It is made up of bones, tendons, small muscles, joint cartilage, ligaments, nerves, and blood vessels, all of which are covered by a thin layer of skin beneath which there is virtually no fat. A normal hand should be bony in appearance, with the tendons on the back of the hand clearly visible when the fingers are extended. The hand should never be puffed or swollen, and any impairment of flexion would signify a basic disturbance of physiology.

As for the face, it should be relaxed, with tiny folds in the skin. Eyelids should lie flat against the cheekbone and the rim of the skull's orbit, neither sunken nor bulged forward. Eyelids are marvelous clinical indicators of vitamin, mineral, and fluid balance.

The cheeks, even in youth, must have tiny wrinkles. As maturity is reached, there is a gradual transition toward increasingly deepening folds. In my clinical experience in northeast Texas between 1962 and 1972, hundreds of my patients had abnormally puffed eyelids and puffed cheeks. Because the persons were swollen, I particularly noticed that tiny wrinkles were absent from their cheeks, which were prominent, bulging, and glistening. This was a significant deviation that will be discussed in more detail in another chapter.

What about the feet and ankles? As with the hands, they should appear almost bony, because they are made of the same basic structures. When the toes are lifted, the same tiny wrinkles should appear on top of the feet as are seen on the back of the normal hand and the cheeks. The skin should be neither puffed nor tight, but loose, pliable, and relaxed.

Simple motor exercises also provide valuable diagnostic data. Early in my treatment of patients with crippled hands I devised a test to determine the extent of their disability. Eventually I came to use the test with all of my patients as a clinical method of screening them for a long-standing need for B$_6$. The Quick Early Warning (QEW) test could lead to early diagnosis and successful treatment, or prevention, of a number of diseases that heretofore have not been suspected of being related to the two joints of the fingers. It is simplicity itself and can be administered in seconds. A person may give it to himself. The reader of this book may test himself without interrupting the reading of these words.

The QEW test consists of this: Hold the hands out with the palms up. Flatten the palms and fingers and keep the wrists straight. This should leave a straight line from the tip of the longest finger to the elbow. Now flex the fingers at the two outer (distal and proximal interphalangeal) joints only, leaving the knuckle (metacarpophalangeal) joints straight with the wrist. By flexing the two outer joints, bring the fingers firmly down to the palms at the metacarpophalangeal crease, to use the anatomical description. The knuckle joint that connects the finger bones to the hand bone must remain straight and unflexed during this test.

It must be emphasized, as I have found necessary to caution my patients, that the knuckle joints must be kept straight. The person taking the test must *not* make a fist. Only the two joints of each finger are to be flexed, and fingertips must touch the palm. (See Fig. 1.)

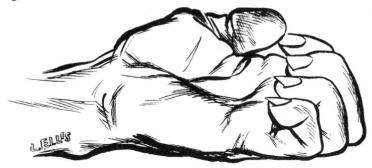

Fig. 1. The Quick Early Warning (QEW) Test

If any one of these sixteen joints, representing the two outer joints of each of the four fingers on each hand, cannot be flexed completely and without pain—barring old fractures, other injuries, and infections—it is probable that one has a need for an increased amount of vitamin B_6. A perfectly healthy person should be able to run through this test readily. But, conversely, capably performing the QEW test without difficulty or pain does not necessarily rule out a need at the cellular, or preclinical, level. Based on my observations and studies with approximately five thousand patients on B_6 therapy, I would doubt that a great many Americans are completely free of some degree of B_6 deficiency.

The Sleeping Giant of Nutrition | 2

Like an iceberg in foggy, uncharted Antarctic waters, vitamin B_6 was a long time emerging from scientific obscurity. Even after the laboratory had assigned it a valid, but sometimes indefinite, role in human nutrition, it remained for years a stepchild of modern medicine—not unwanted, perhaps, but both overlooked and undervalued. Today its image is still blurred in medical circles, and even more so in the public mind, a fact that was forcibly driven home to me on reading this dictionary definition of pyridoxine: "A complex pyridine compound, one of the B complex vitamins, found in various foods and prepared synthetically, usually as the hydrochloride: known to prevent nutritional dermatitis in rats: also called B_6."[1]

Vitamin B_6 has come a long way from its only known role of preventing nutritional dermatitis in rats, which was proved about forty years ago, but it has not yet fixed itself in the public mind as to its other vital contributions. It still faces a steep climb to the point where it can be said that the medical profession has accepted it as a routine daily medication.

Yet behind that terse dictionary entry lies a rich history of a nutrient that stretches back to the dawn of vitamin research, back at least to the first work done with the B-complex vitamins, for vitamin B_6, like that shrouded Antarctic iceberg, was for a long time a sleeping giant. And in the early years of vitamin research the giant was also invisible.

Because all vitamins of the B complex are intimately tied to each other in their histories, the story of B_6 necessarily begins with the discovery of vitamin B, as B_1 was then known. To a large extent, vitamin B_6 could not be discovered until others were discovered. Its discovery was an offshoot, or windfall, of research aimed at finding other nutrients. It had to wait its turn. For this reason the history of B_6 is also the history of those B vitamins sought before it was found. B_1, or thiamine, is the antiberiberi specific. The first discovery of a beriberi cure apparently came in 1897 in a Java hospital when the Dutch physician Christiaan Eykman fed experimental chickens polished rice. They got beriberi. He cured the disorder by then feeding them unhusked rice, but unfortunately his findings were published only in Dutch and did not become widely known. Subsequently, in 1909, two British scientists, Henry Fraser and Ambrose Stanton, conducted similar studies that showed beriberi was caused by a deficiency in the diet.

The vitamin B story unfolded with a major chapter in 1912 when Casimir Funk (1884–1967), a Polish-born biochemist doing research in London, established that polished rice caused a beriberilike disease in pigeons. Next, from 836 pounds of unpolished rice, he separated the antiberiberi factor, which subsequently became known as vitamin B, or thiamine. He also accomplished another remarkable feat: he separated nicotinic acid from unpolished rice—but he didn't realize that it was the antipellagra factor, thereby postponing its use for more than a quarter of a century.* It was Funk who proposed, that same year, the "vitamine hypothesis": the idea that the deficiency diseases beriberi, scurvy, and possibly pellagra and rickets, were caused by the absence of a specific chemical substance from the diet. He also gave the world the name *vitamine*, later shortened to *vitamin*, because he thought that he had discovered a protein, or amino acid, in-

---

* In 1972 Dr. Samuel Lepkovsky, a scientist we will be meeting subsequently in these pages, told me: "Casimir Funk once visited me and told me that he isolated nicotinic acid and that he suspected it was a vitamin."

stead. But in discovering the nutrient that was to become B_1, Funk did not synthesize it.

From the time that Funk discovered B_1 in rice polishings, much scientific attention was thereafter focused on the treatment and prevention of pellagra, a debilitating disease that ravaged the American South and other poor regions of the world. Pellagra, a scourging Goliath that had been recognized as a specific disorder as early as 1735 in Spain and later in Italy with a word meaning "rough skin," now drew the concentrated attention of scientists the world over, especially in the United States, where it had reached epidemic proportions as a mass disabler that killed. Pellagra hovered like a dark specter over the American rural South, where, as in the afflicted regions of Europe, the poor subsisted on diets consisting mainly of corn. In the early twentieth century as many as 170,000 new cases appeared there annually.

In 1915 the scientist who was to become the major hero of the pellagra war went into the field for the U.S. Public Health Service to study conditions in the South. He was Dr. Joseph Goldberger, who had come to the United States from Hungary as a small child.

Observing both patients and staff members of state asylums in South Carolina, Georgia, and Mississippi, Goldberger established that pellagra was a deficiency disease. This was no small accomplishment, for no one knew its etiology or cause, and at the time, in fact, there were several conflicting theories. But Goldberger noted that the patients developed pellagra, while staff members of the asylums did not. Logically, he attributed this difference to the fact that the patients, fed cereals, did not eat the milk, meat, and eggs that the doctors and nurses did. Correctly, he concluded that pellagra was a disease of dietary deficiency, but he related it to a lack of protein in the daily diet.

In order to prove that pellagra was not a contagious disease, Goldberger subjected his own body—and the bodies of his associates, including his wife—to injections of excrement, nasal mucus, and scale from the pellagra sufferers. He—and the others—remained free of pellagra, thereby demonstrating his proof dramatically. He delivered his report to the Southern Medical Association in Atlanta, Georgia, on November 13, 1916.

The contagion theory eliminated, he then could concentrate on finding the antipellagra specific that he knew was in food. He wasted no effort. Subsequently, he brought about swift recoveries by using yeast, beef, and milk to supplement the regular diets of patients who had come down with pellagra. Studying "blacktongue" in dogs, he accurately concluded that it was the same as pellagra in human brings. And liver extract both cured beriberi and prevented blacktongue in dogs. Thus, liver extract had in it both the antiberiberi and the antipellagra factors. But what, precisely, were they? Tragically, Goldberger was never to learn. He died of cancer in 1929. His pioneer work was destined to be finished by others in the decade to follow.

The scientific world, in both Europe and the United States, was in ferment during the late nineteen twenties. In 1927 the British Committee on Accessory Food Factors recognized two separate components of the vitamin B complex: vitamin B_1, the antineuritic, antiberiberi factor, and vitamin B_2, then considered to be the antipellagra factor and, although yet to be isolated, believed to be the only other factor in what is now termed the B complex.

From the vantage point of nearly a half century afterward it is easy for us to see that the term "vitamin B_2" actually was a large umbrella that covered a number of B-complex vitamins besides the antipellagra factor. This meant that in addition to niacin, which was later accepted as the antipellagra factor they were seeking, vitamin B_2 at the time included, with others, riboflavin as well as vitamin B_6. Thus, our sleeping giant remained well concealed, with only two factors known to exist in the richly populated B-complex world: There was B_1, the antineuritic or antiberiberi factor, and then there was B_2—which, in effect, meant everything else that we now know to be in the group. How were scientists to know, at that stage of their investigations, that isolating the B vitamins was to be as complicated—and as rewarding —as sorting out rare, twinkling gems from an ancient family jewel case? It was as if the label of the jewel chest had read *Rubies* but on opening it one discovered, along with rubies, many other kinds of gems, including diamonds, emeralds, and opals.

But because the other substances were not at first suspected to be in the jewel case labeled "B_2," a search through the medical literature of the time is frequently confusing to the present-day doctor, as well as the general reader. After a time one may not be certain what one is reading, as articles refer to the unknown "other" fraction of the B world variously as vitamin B_2, P-P (pellagra-preventive), and vitamin G.

This was the general situation, then, in the late twenties when Dr. Paul György, a young professor of pediatrics at Heidelberg University, became interested in dermatological conditions of infants, a concern that was to lead him down a network of investigatory trails—and to a major role in the discoveries of three of the B-complex vitamins: riboflavin (vitamin B_2), biotin, and pyridoxine (vitamin B_6).

György, a native of Hungary, was awarded his M.D. degree at the University of Budapest in 1915, in time to serve in the Austro-Hungarian army as a medical officer during World War I. In 1920 he was appointed professor of pediatrics at Heidelberg University, where he began his vitamin research and where he taught until 1933.

It is interesting to note, since the research on vitamin B_6 was so very much an international effort involving many laboratories, that György during this fertile period of research was on the faculties of three universities in different countries: first Heidelberg, then Cambridge University in England for two years, and, beginning in 1935, Western Reserve University in Cleveland, Ohio. By the time he had gone to the University of Pennsylvania in 1944, where at this writing he is professor emeritus and an active consultant, he had completed the bulk of his work on these three vitamins.

György first attempted to study the dermatological conditions experimentally by using various rations on rats.[2] He was especially interested in seborrhoid dermatitis—an inflammation resulting in abnormally oily, scaly skin—and acrodynia. In acrodynia, as observed in the laboratory, scaly sores appeared on the tails, ears, and paws of the experimental rats.

Looking back on those earlier days of vitamin research, when the study of nutrition was practically in its infancy, one finds a striking contrast with today's streamlined, microbiological tests that give results often within hours. In the twenties, when scientists were laying the foundations that would vitally benefit their successors, patience seemed a much greater virtue than it is today. It generally took much longer to assay chemically substances used in feeding studies. György, for instance, labored twelve years before publishing his first scientific paper on biotin.

Although a story of vitamin research in those years reads like a roll call of Nobel Prize winners or a Who's Who in Science, funds and assistants were not always easily come by. Research often meant personal involvement of one's family as well. During a 1970 visit of the Györgys to my Texas ranch, Margaret György described to me those days of the twenties and thirties. "It's not like it used to be," she said. "Back then I fed the rats for his experiments. Now they have people who do that."

Essentially, in the isolation and identification of vitamin B_2 (riboflavin), there were three steps that also led to the discovery of B_6. These were the attempts to ascertain the nature of the fluorescent material that was found in milk whey, to isolate material from milk whey that is an essential dietary factor for the rat (initially designated as vitamin B_2), and the isolation of the coenzyme of the "old yellow enzyme," as it was called, from red cells.

The three directions, or definite lines of investigation, that broadened out of the original search led, eventually, to the discovery of three different vitamins. The first pertained to "egg white injury," a deficiency condition that was produced in rats limited to a ration of dry, uncooked egg white as the only source of protein. A raw-egg-white diet, it was learned, caused very severe generalized scaly dermatitis and loss of weight, ending in death. To pin down the precise mechanism György worked from 1929 until 1940 on this aspect of the original undertaking, finally discovering biotin by proving that something in uncooked egg white bound it so that it was unavailable to the animal. Cooked, the egg white allowed absorption of the essential biotin, the known yeast-growth-promoting factor.

Dr. Vincent du Vigneaud, who was to win the Nobel Prize in Chemistry in 1955 for discovering a process for making synthetic hormones, was then professor of biochemistry at the Cornell School of Medicine and was György's chemical collaborator in the studies. Biotin was subsequently established as important to all living organisms.

A personal anecdote will illustrate, perhaps, to some extent the breadth of György's twelve-year search for biotin, as well as the depth of my own ignorance on the subject when Dr. György visited me in Texas in the spring of 1970.

In company with my foreman I was driving Dr. György over my ranch. Stopping in a pasture I had especially cultivated for my herd of Brahman cattle, of which I was most proud, I jumped from the car to pull up a handful of crimson clover plants. I blew off the dirt from the legumes to display them to the distinguished scientist.

"What is he doing?" Dr. György asked my ranch foreman.

"He wants to show you the nodules on the roots of the clover," said the foreman. By then I was back in the car. The foreman continued, "It's oxygen."

"No," I corrected the foreman, "it's not oxygen—it's nitrogen in the nodules!"

"Yes. I know," said Dr. György in his fascinating Hungarian accent. "Biotin binds it there."

Along with his other experiments during his long work, he had turned his cellar into a kind of home laboratory in which he had studied various plants, patiently deepening his understanding of the functions of biotin.

The second study grew out of the original dermatological problem and related to the isolation of vitamin B$_2$, which, as we have seen, was at first believed to be only one other substance that was not B$_1$ in the B complex. His collaborators in these investigations were two of Europe's leading scientists, Professor Richard Kuhn and Dr. Theodor Wagner-Jauregg. Kuhn, of the chemistry department at Heidelberg University, subsequently won the Nobel Prize in Chemistry, in 1938, for his work on carotenoids and vitamins. Tragically, Kuhn and other Germans were forced by the Nazis, under threat of violence, to decline all Nobel prizes. Hitler's anger had been provoked in 1936 when Carl von Ossietzky, a pacifist and anti-Nazi in prison at the time, had been awarded the Nobel Peace Prize. Thereafter, Hitler forbade any German to accept the most prestigious international award.

György did the "rat work" in the B$_2$ project that involved feeding the rats a purified supplemented diet containing cod-liver oil, for vitamins A and D, and an alcoholic extract of what was the source of vitamin B_1 (thiamine). The chemist, Wagner-Jauregg, separated the fractions; György observed the growth of the rats. The rats were tested over periods of three to four weeks each, very time-consuming in comparison to today's microbiological tests that may be done in hours.

As Wagner-Jauregg prepared a number of concentrates from cow's milk in order to isolate the various fractions chemically, György observed the growth of the rats. Progress was made when Wagner-Jauregg noted that the active concentrates were colored, characterized by an intensive *green-yellow fluorescence* that existed in direct proportion to the biological effects. The end of the long search seemed near. As a working hypothesis they identified the long-sought B_2 with the yellow-green fluorescence. Accordingly, the chemist further refined the concentrates until they became more and more colored, greener and greener.

But one day, carefully observing the rats, György notified Wagner-Jauregg that something had gone wrong. The rats were not growing. In the purifying procedure something essential had been taken out—the vitamin B_2 they had been seeking, apparently. The green-yellow fluorescence, then, was not what they had hoped it would be. They had been wrong in identifying B_2 with color alone. It was not green after all. The disappointed Wagner-Jauregg, in despair at the failure of the working hypothesis and, it seemed, of the entire experiment, discussed it with György. In the discussion that followed, György showed that by supplementation with a specially prepared yeast concentrate the biological activity of the colored preparation could be restored. Wagner-Jauregg reworked the experiment, backtracking over the just-traveled trail, so to speak, by adding fractions that had already been eliminated.

In this way vitamin B_2 was isolated by chemists Kuhn and Wagner-Jauregg, with György as a collaborator, as the pure crystalline yellow compound from milk whey. They first called it *lactoflavin* but later it acquired the name *riboflavin*.

The discovery of riboflavin was a breakthrough, for the nutrient bridged the gap between an essential nutrient and cell enzymes and cellular metabolism. It was the first vitamin to be recognized as a part of an enzyme system. This, in biochemical research, represented a special milestone, for since then water-soluble vitamins have been found to be essential parts of enzyme systems.

The structure of riboflavin was established by Richard Kuhn, and it was synthesized by both Kuhn and Paul Karrer. The Swiss scientist Karrer was destined to receive the Nobel Prize in Chemistry in 1937 for his studies of carotenoids, flavins, and vitamins A and B.

Ironically, the antipellagra factor, which vitamin B$_2$ was expected to be, was yet to be found. Riboflavin, or B$_2$, definitely was an essential vitamin, but it would not specifically cure pellagra. The discovery was but an example of serendipity that would characterize the B-complex research story for years. Search for one precious gem turned up, instead, another, but the finding of one helped lead to another.

The P-P, or pellagra-preventive, hunt continued unabated. Now György had two B-complex vitamins in pure form that he could use in tracking down his internationally sought quarry. In 1933 crystalline thiamine or B$_1$ had become available; now he had riboflavin as well. These were his major keys. Again, he returned to his experimental rats to run further feeding experiments. He placed the rats on a diet lacking the whole vitamin B complex but supplemented with required amounts of thiamine and riboflavin, the only two known B vitamins. In this way he could determine if there were any other essential members of the B family.

After a few weeks on this diet the young rats showed a reduced rate of growth and developed scaly sores, or dermatitis, that was most pronounced on the peripheral parts of the body, such as the tail, paws, ears, and snout. There also was an accompanying edema, or swelling of the structures involved in the sores. This apparently minor condition was of great importance in distinguishing the disorder from dermatitis caused by a diet deficient in certain polyunsaturated fats.

The cutaneous lesions somewhat resembled those found on human beings suffering from pellagra, which inspired György to call the condition he had induced in rats "pellagra-like" but "without prejudice as to their identity or nonidentity with human pellagra." Thus György established that vitamin B_2 was not a single vitamin but a complex in itself.

At the time, other investigators had already claimed the names B_3, B_4, B_5, as well as Y, for substances they believed to be vitamins. Therefore, György skipped these and labeled his "rat pellagra" vitamin B_6. Vitamin B_3 was the pellagra-preventive, later to be labeled nicotinic acid or niacin. Subsequent discussion formulated the view that B_4 and B_5 were not vitamins but other substances; for this reason, at present there are no such vitamins as B_4 and B_5—they turned out to be "dud experiments."

Although György had made the discovery, much hard work remained to be done to prove definitely that his claimed vitamin B_6 actually existed as a separate nutrient. For the next two years, from 1935 to 1937, investigations by a number of scientists established the distinction between riboflavin and B_6, as well as Goldberger's P-P factor. This work, participated in by György, Dr. Conrad A. Elvehjem, an instructor at the Agricultural College of the University of Wisconsin, and others, "definitely established the separate existence of these three members of the vitamin B complex," in the words of György. (In 1937 Elvehjem determined that nicotinic acid, or niacin, was the P-P factor that researchers had been intensively seeking since Goldberger's work on pellagra in 1916.) As one result of this differentiation, the designation "pellagra-like dermatitis" of vitamin B_6 deficiency was changed to "rat acrodynia," but without any reference to human acrodynia.

The next step was to isolate the pure crystalline vitamin B_6, which was to be found in liver and yeast. György was but one of many who were strenuously laboring to isolate the vitamin. I had the privilege of discussing this period with Dr. Samuel Lepkovsky, one of the scientists involved, when I visited San Francisco in 1972. Lepkovsky, Polish-born like Funk (and who knew Funk), came to the United States with his parents when he was six years old, when the family settled in Wisconsin. As we discussed this earlier period, Lepkovsky recalled György's preparing a crude fraction containing the nutrient that would relieve rat acrodynia, which was reported in the scientific literature.

"Paul György laid the foundation for all of this work [with pyridoxine] and then the race was on between Richard Kuhn of the I. G. Farben Company [in Germany], the Merck Company in this country, and I was the dark horse. I learned that Paul and I had about reached the same place, and I wrote him and urged him to send in his paper because I had isolated the pure compound."

And then Samuel Lepkovsky added something that I will never forget: "Research by itself is worthwhile without seeking the honor of who is first."

This was in 1938 when the goal was in sight for several of the investigators, and it was early that year that Lepkovsky, in a warm gesture not often experienced in the highly competitive world of scientific research, advised György that he and another scientist, J. C. Keresztesy, were ready to submit, independently of each other, their own papers for publication. This enabled György, now aware of the urgency, to submit his own publication in time. Lepkovsky's gesture was one that György never forgot.

Lepkovsky, then, was the first to report the isolation of pure crystalline B$_6$ from liver and yeast, in an article in the American journal *Science* in 1938, just four years after its discovery by György. The same year, slightly later, others, including György, reported its isolation independently of Lepkovsky, in American, German, and Japanese scientific journals.

Within a year, American researchers Stanton A. Harris and Karl Folkers of Merck and Company's research laboratory, writing in the *Journal of the American Chemical Society* (April 14, 1939), and Germans Richard Kuhn, K. Westphal, G. Wendt, and O. Westphal, in *Naturwissenschaften*, had made clear the exact chemical structure of vitamin B$_6$, as shown in Figure 2.

György proposed the term *pyridoxine* for the compound be-

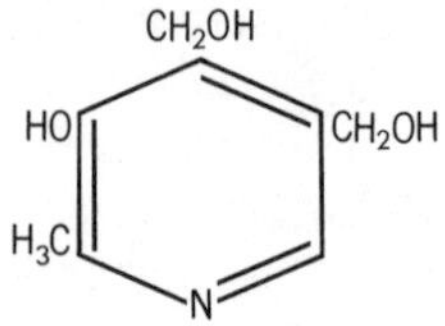

Fig. 2. Pyridoxine

cause it contained the pyridine ring, as shown here. The label has received general acceptance. Thus, as the father of vitamin B_6, Paul György discovered it, independently isolated it, and, finally, named it pyridoxine, thus closing out what he was later to classify as "one of the most intriguing chapters in the rapid development of vitamin research."[3] It is no small wonder that thereafter the nutrient was to have his stamp on it, although scores of other researchers were to be connected intimately with research on it.

At this stage, immediately after its discovery, isolation, and synthesis, pyridoxine, or vitamin B_6, was in the curious position of being, at least temporarily, a glamour vitamin but with its proved usefulness limited to the relief of rat acrodynia. And although some brief clinical work was done with it, this is essentially the way it was to remain for more than a decade.

However, the clinical work appeared promising and seemed to assure a future for the vitamin. By June 10, 1939, less than two months after its synthesis, three doctors in Birmingham, Alabama, writing in the *Journal of the American Medical Association,* reported what apparently was its first human use. The doctors—Tom Douglas Spies, another pioneer in the pellagra war, William B. Bean, and William F. Ashe—announced dramatic, twenty-four-hour recoveries of four patients after having been treated with pure vitamin B_6 at the Hillman Hospital in Birmingham. Earlier, the four persons had been treated for pellagra and beriberi, caused respectively by deficiencies of niacin and thiamine. However, the patients soon returned to their old inadequate diets, again developing their old symptoms. This time, however, they were each given 50 milligrams of pure synthetic vitamin B_6. Both doctors and patients were astounded when all the symptoms disappeared within twenty-four hours. Before treatment, one man had been unable to walk more than a few steps. The day after he was injected with B_6 he walked two miles without fatigue![4]

Spies, who later, near the end of his career, was to receive the Distinguished Service Award of the American Medical Association, was a clinical pioneer in treating pellagra and other deficiency diseases following the discovery and synthesis of niacin as the P-P specific. In 1940 Spies reported additional remarkable changes effected by B_6 therapy. Speaking at the 100th annual meeting of the Illinois State Medical Society, Spies told of patients suffering from Parkinson's disease who responded within a few minutes after intravenous injections. Parkinson's disease, a shaking palsy marked by muscular weakness, stiffness, and pain, was a severe and lingering disease that had hitherto been considered more or less hopeless. Spies and his associate William B. Bean treated eleven cases of Parkinsonism that had existed for at least four years. Eight of the cases were arteriosclerotic and three were post-encephalitic. Their best results came with the three patients who had had encephalitis, these showing improvement a few minutes after injection. Tremors and rigidity decreased so that the patients could walk without their customary stiffness.

Two of the arteriosclerotic patients showed definite improvement, five were unchanged, and one was considerably worse.

Dr. Spies also reported that similar results with B_6 therapy with Parkinsonism patients had been communicated to him by Dr. Norman H. Jolliffe of the New York University College of Medicine.[5] These reports, however, soon faded away without inspiring any widespread, intensive clinical activity related to B_6.

It was at this point, when clinical interest seemed to be fading, that microbiological research entered the picture. In 1942 a brilliant biochemist at the University of Texas, Dr. Esmond E. Snell, still in his twenties, established the existence of two other forms of vitamin B_6—pyridoxal and pyridoxamine. Snell found that the three forms existed in nature in plants and that there was a difference in the rate of growth of certain bacteria, depending on which one of the three forms was present. He also proved that, once taken into the human body, these combine with phosphate to form pyridoxal phosphate, which from that point on is the reactive principle of B_6. It is this coenzyme that speeds up and stimulates the necessary biochemical reactions in human metabolism.

Thus vitamin B_6 became known as a subgroup of the vitamin B_2 complex, with pyridoxine, pyridoxal, and pyridoxamine as its particular chemical representatives. Subsequently it was found to be distributed widely in both animal and plant products, usually as pyridoxine in plants and seeds, as pyridoxal and pyridoxamine in animal products. It was found most abundantly in whole-grain cereals, fish, milk, eggs, vegetables, and yeast. While pyridoxine seemed stable to heat, pyridoxal and pyridoxamine could be partially destroyed by cooking, and all forms were sensitive to light and vigorous oxidation. In fact, all of the B vitamins are water-soluble, and the longer that green vegetables are boiled, the less food value they have. Among the B_6-rich foods that can be eaten uncooked are brewers yeast, wheat germ, bananas, pecans, and avocados. By chemical analysis a banana has been found to be about five times richer in vitamin B_6, gram for gram, than any other fruit.

Close on the heels of Snell's discovery, Samuel Lepkovsky (who earlier had isolated B_6) and associates, working at the University of California at Berkeley and the California Institute of Technology at Pasadena, in 1943 reported the isolation of xanthurenic acid (XA) from the urine of pyridoxine-deficient rats. Xanthurenic acid was shown to be an abnormal metabolite of the amino acid tryptophan and related to vitamin B_6 deficiency. When pyridoxine was added to the diet, xanthurenic acid immediately disappeared from the urine. Thus, xanthurenic acid was recognized as an indication of metabolic derangement as the result of inadequate pyridoxine levels.[6]

This work led to the development of a valuable diagnostic tool that was to see extensive use in the years ahead—the tryptophan load test. If tryptophan is not metabolized normally, xanthurenic acid, among others, will be excreted in the urine. Following the work of Lepkovsky's group, the test became a common one to determine the B_6 levels in both man and experimental animals.[7]

In the years that followed, despite the laboratory findings and the beginning work of Spies with human beings, B_6 seemed to go through a period of doldrums with few uses found for it clinically. In the words of discoverer György, "with all the rich history of vitamin B_6, approximately twenty years passed before its requirement by the human organism had been definitely established and recognized."[8] One of the reasons for this was the disrupting effect of World War II, which conscripted the energies and talents of scientists around the world and kept doctors overworked merely taking care of their patients, pre-empting further proper clinical investigations. By the time the war was over, medical interest had been refocused on other, more glamorous fields. It was as if B_6 had been left by the wayside as new wonder drugs competed among each other for the spotlight.

Excluding the Spies episodes, it was 1952 before the first evidence came that B_6 was essential to man. That year an excessively heated commercial milk formula caused convulsions in infants. It was subsequently proved that naturally occurring vitamin B_6 in the formula was destroyed by heat to the point where a resulting deficiency caused serious impairment of brain function.

The story began in little Harrison, Arkansas, a county-seat town in the Ozarks, when a mother telephoned Dr. William P. Barron that her baby was having a convulsion. The baby, shaking all over, had turned blue. Dr. Barron rushed to the home and methodically examined the baby but found no evidence of serious disease. Hospitalizing the baby, he ordered all diagnostic tests that might cast light: X rays, blood, urine, and spinal-fluid studies. All tests returned "negative," indicating that the baby was healthy. But the convulsions continued.

In the hospital the baby was fed a whole-milk-and-sugar formula instead of the commercial formula he had been getting. By the third day of hospitalization the baby had but one seizure. By the fourth day his convulsions had ended. What had changed to improve the baby's condition? There seemed to be no clues, nothing to go on. But soon, as similar cases came into that and other hospitals, a pattern began to appear. The babies were mainly from four to sixteen weeks old, they were convulsing, and they were on the same commercial formula. When their formulas were changed, the convulsions disappeared.

Dr. Barron and others, including Dr. B. P. Briggs of Little Rock and Dr. J. O. Cooper of El Dorado, reported their observations to the State Health Department in Little Rock.

Although cases were reported in various parts of the country, a concentration of them was channeled to the State Health Department in Little Rock, where the milk formula had become suspect. By May 12, 1953, the matter had reached the American Medical Association's Council on Foods and Nutrition, which sought details from the University of Arkansas School of Medicine in Little Rock. Dr. Katharine Dodd, professor of pediatrics, personally went through the records of the cases handled there, copied them in longhand, and dispatched them to Chicago. At the same time Dr. Johan Eliot, pediatric consultant to the Arkansas State Health Department, one of the first to suspect a connection between formula and the convulsions, sent the AMA his records, collected from parts of Texas as well as Arkansas. Further evidence was contributed by Dr. David B. Coursin of Lancaster, Pennsylvania.

Within forty-eight hours the council had collected enough evidence to implicate the formula definitely. The manufacturer was notified. The company voluntarily took the formula off the market. By May 22 all of the milk had been removed from all of the stores in the United States.[9]

In the process of pinning down the flaw in the formula, it was learned that the company had made changes in its product some time earlier. It had substituted a new type of fat, and the formula had been heated more than previously. Later investigators were to blame excessive heating for the B_6 deficiency of the formula.

I discussed this with L. J. Filer, M.D., Ph.D., now professor of pediatrics at the University of Iowa School of Medicine, and he told me, "O. L. Kline, because of some work he had done with rats, suspected that the convulsions were caused by inadequate B_6, and I did the assay on the milk that determined this."

Subsequently Coursin, director of research at St. Joseph's Hospital in Lancaster, Pennsylvania, proved, by use of an electroencephalogram during a baby's convulsions, that B_6 injections would stop convulsions and would prevent subsequent ones. Thus it was learned that naturally occurring B_6 could be destroyed by heat to a point where the resulting dietary deficiency caused serious impairment of brain function.

In other hospitals and clinics it was learned that B_6 would also relieve neuritis in the arms, legs, hands, and feet of tuberculosis patients who were treated with certain drugs. The drug isoniazid, used in treating tuberculosis, induced a B_6 deficiency by combining with the active form of the vitamin, pyridoxal phosphate, and causing its elimination in the urine.[10] For this reason, tuberculosis sanitariums began using large amounts of B₆ to counteract the destruction by the drug antagonists.

Other investigators revealed a relationship between an increased need for B₆ and mental retardation. Convulsive seizures occurred in children who were mentally retarded; these convulsions could be eliminated by increased amounts of B₆. In another area, radiologists used B₆ to some extent in an effort to relieve nausea associated with deep X-ray therapy in the treatment of cancer. Meanwhile, obstetricians claimed some success in treating nausea of pregnancy with B₆, and the vitamin was found useful in relieving a rare type of anemia in which red blood cells were too small. This was not the usual iron-deficiency anemia; it apparently resulted from a defective hereditary factor that was responsive to B₆.[11] One other isolated clinical experience had been the successful treatment of a peculiar type of photosensitivity, a rare condition characterized by intolerance to sunlight and severe sunburn with very little exposure.

Summarizing the work of these decades, Paul György has written that "the history of vitamin B₆ is a further proof that success usually is preceded by trials, tribulations, and recurrent disappointment. The most helpful factor, apart from perseverance and timeliness of the line of research, is the deliberate recognition of a principle that is paramount in scientific research; it is often almost beyond our control, and touches closely on intuition. It is Walter B. Cannon's 'serendipity.' "[12] It was an apt characterization of B₆ history, and on the basis of my own experiences with the vitamin, I would agree with a *Journal of the American Medical Association* editorial on another subject that, "Apparently, unlike lightning, serendipity can strike more than once in the same place, and, as distinct from the former, it illuminates without destroying."[13]

This, basically, was the sum of the rich history of vitamin B₆ when I first became interested in the nutrient in 1961. Needless to say, I was not then aware of what I have written in this chapter. I had not read on the subject to any extent. Nor was I then aware of the early clinical work of Dr. Spies. Although evidence was already building up in the laboratory that pointed to the dangers of B_6 deficiency, it was far from common knowledge among doctors—as it still is—and in 1961 there was a prevalent concept that B_6 deficiency did not exist in the United States.

Prior to that time it appeared that human beings who responded to B_6 had rare and unusual disease conditions, and these were primarily limited to clinical findings in infants who had convulsed following use of a defective milk formula and in tubercular patients who developed peripheral neuritis after treatment with drug antagonists.

Although others, especially in the laboratory, were undoubtedly working on various aspects of B_6 research at the time, I was unaware of their efforts in 1961 when I became involved in clinical research in a way that can only be termed serendipitous. My interest in this field came in a rather roundabout, but logical, fashion as the result of my heightened concern over heart disease in my patients. By the early nineteen sixties I, like many other physicians, had had a number of patients killed by heart attacks. I soon grew accustomed to peeping through oxygen tents at ghastly pale patients in shock, with cold, clammy sweat on their faces, and I became determined to exert every effort I could to find some way to change this trend that, both nationally and in my own practice, was becoming an epidemic.

At the time, many researchers believed they had found the major cause of heart disease. They thought it was cholesterol, and the point seemed substantiated by the prominent role of saturated fats in the American diet. But the controversy was far from being one-sided. A bombardment of medical claims bolstered first one side, then the other. In 1961 when I decided to pursue a preventive program with my patients the issue was red-hot, and it fanned higher with each new medical communiqué.

Certainly it seemed a logical, sensible approach to cut down drastically on patients' intake of saturated fats. Nothing alters a person's body more than the food he eats. Food has both direct and indirect bearing on one's health, depending on the quality, quantity, and kind of food. Thus the role of fat metabolism was a logical factor to consider in heart disease, for the American diet was composed of nearly 50 percent fats.

Having read the work of Dr. Ancel Keys, I began a study of

the American diet. Dr. Keys was director of the Laboratory of Physiological Hygiene at the University of Minnesota. He was the man for whom the famed K-ration of World War II was named. His primary interest was fat and cholesterol.

After analyzing several diets, I selected a low-fat diet developed by Dr. Lester M. Morrison of the College of Medical Evangelists in Los Angeles. Dr. Morrison had reported in the *Journal of the American Medical Association* that he had used the diet to treat successfully victims of coronary thrombosis.[14] Essentially the diet substituted lean meat for fat meat and suggested that vegetables and fruits be increased. Vegetable oils were used for cooking instead of saturated fats of animal origin. Although the diet was presumed to be balanced in minerals and vitamins, its main appeal to me at that time was that it would relieve the body of ingesting the usual high-fat diet at which cardiologists were pointing the finger of blame.

My first patient on the Morrison diet became, in a way, my first patient in what was ultimately to be my clinical work with B₆. He was a tall, ruddy-faced, 210-pound oilfield worker. At fifty-five he outwardly appeared to be in the best of health. He hadn't been in a doctor's office in five years. But that day he didn't know whether he was, as he expressed it, "sick or crazy." His hands and arms tingled; the symptoms had been bothering him for months. Sometimes, he complained, it felt as if "waves of electricity" were going up and down his arms and into his chest. When I began my diagnostic questions he remembered that he had cramps in his legs after going to bed. As I examined his hands, the veins and tendons were not visible on the backs of his hands, suggesting a slight edema, but at the time I did not assign much significance to it.

He had been consuming a high-cholesterol diet. He seemed to be an ideal candidate for the low-fat Morrison diet. I gave him a printed sheet with instructions and told him to return in two weeks. But his symptoms piqued my curiosity, and I began asking other patients if their hands tingled or if their leg muscles cramped at night. Each went on the Morrison diet.

When the oilfield worker returned, his old symptoms were gone, but now he had pain in the shoulders and elbows. The low-fat diet had helped, but it hadn't restored him to complete health. On his third visit, though, he reported a change that impressed both of us. He had lost eight pounds, without attempting to do so, and he had lost three inches off his waistline! Yet he had not cut down on his food intake, for I had not emphasized calories or the measuring of food. It was more important to me to secure the full cooperation of my patients in eating the particular types of food that the Morrison diet recommended.

Evidence accumulated swiftly. A forty-year-old woman I had known since high school, whose deep freezer was filled with pork sausage, ham, and bacon, complained of muscle spasms in her feet at night that brought tears to her eyes. After thirty-six hours on the Morrison diet, she became free of her symptoms. A seventy-three-year-old farm woman, suffering from severe tingling, cramps, fainting, vertigo, and painful elbows and shoulders, came in with a serum cholesterol level of 311 milligrams percent—quite high. (The normal is from 150 to 250 milligrams.) On the Morrison diet, her tingling paresthesias, muscle spasms, fainting, and vertigo vanished, and the elbow-shoulder pain gradually improved.

After one office visit she blurted out: "If I knew how to play a piano, I could play it!"

She showed what she meant by vigorously flexing her fingers back and forth rapidly, as a pianist might warm up for the evening's concert.

"You see, I can move my fingers better," she said. "I couldn't do that before I went on the diet."

Her words intrigued me for long afterward. Why did her fingers move better? *How* did they move better? She had been taken off her saturated fats, but there was more involved than merely an absence of fats. She, as well as the others, was getting something extra in her diet, something she hadn't been getting before. What positive factor was it that had restored her finger function almost overnight? The answers to these questions clearly lay in the diet, but how could the specific factor be pinpointed?

The answers were slow in coming. Gradually I realized that the medical profession was blocked from final positive proof that the excessive consumption of saturated fats alone caused coronary thrombosis. Each time the epidemiologists thought they had the solution, somebody like the Eskimo popped up. The Eskimo at that time had little heart disease; yet he ate blubber, probably the diet highest in saturated fats.

By then I also realized that my patients had not been getting balanced diets before and that the Morrison diet was a high-vitamin, high-mineral diet. Frequently they had been eating diets containing more than 50 percent fats. When a person eats the fat from a steak, he gets no minerals, no vitamins, no enzymes, no nutrients—just calories. Fat calories are as "empty" as those in sugar. A diet composed of 50 percent fat means that half of the diet provides no proper nutrition.[15] The vitamins, minerals, and other nutrients have to come from the other half of the diet. The fat-eater is as bad off in most ways as the man who expects to get his calories from alcohol alone. When alcohol displaces food, the person develops vitamin deficiencies. The same severe deficiencies may come from burning calories from fat—or sugar —alone. Additionally, a high-fat diet may lead to obesity, for fat must either become energy, human fat, or waste. The arithmetic is simple. There are nine calories to a gram of fat and four to a gram of protein. It doesn't take many servings of fat to add up to a gain in weight.

My first progress in nailing down the specific most beneficial ingredient in the diet came, as often happens with a doctor, through another patient. The man, a bachelor teacher in his sixties, was free of symptoms. He merely came in for a regular physical examination, to make sure he was as healthy as he felt. He was. He seemed to be enjoying such glowing health that I marveled at his suntan, still retained in the depth of winter, and his general appearance. I asked him about his diet. For the past eighteen months, he said, he had been eating pecans every day and cooking with peanut oil, the results of a diet he had heard about. Everything else he ate as he always had. Could he tell a difference? Yes. For forty-five years he had had pain in his knees every night after retiring; now it was gone. He had a stronger grip. His fingers were more limber, more flexible—they were not "stiff or fat."

Again, some dietary factor was at work, and it seemed to be

present in pecans and peanuts. Might not these nuts help other patients?

A few days later a sixty-six-year-old woman, who had been hospitalized for diabetes and chest pain, came in for a follow-up examination. She required fifty units of insulin daily to keep her blood sugar from going too high. I put her on the Morrison diet, with diabetic modifications. I told her to eat peanuts and pecans each day.

In two weeks she had "just a little bit" of chest pain, a great improvement. Her fingers had been hurting; now only one did. They were no longer stiff and she could do her work.

Her case was more than casually interesting. Sixteen years before, she had had a leg amputated above the knee, because of bone cancer. For the past five years she had been on a controlled diabetic diet. Before the Morrison diet she had had tingling of the hands and her one leg cramped for years. Now, after two weeks on the Morrison diet supplemented by pecans and peanuts, those symptoms were gone, and she added, as a lagniappe, "I just feel better than I have felt in years."

Again, why? What, specifically, had changed her health so suddenly? In order to attempt to nail down the particular ingredient that was doing so much good, after much thought I decided to work with the B-complex vitamins. Undoubtedly the patients had been getting B vitamins in the diet, and B-complex deficiencies produced a broad spectrum of disease conditions. I would start by working with five B vitamins: thiamine (B_1), riboflavin (B_2), nicotinic acid (niacin), pantothenic acid, and pyridoxine (B_6). If these vitamins produced the same results that the diet had, then the search would be narrowed down. From that point on, the specific B vitamins could be identified. On the other hand, if these five vitamins did not materially alleviate symptoms, all of them could be ruled out and the search could continue with other nutrients.

In order to have a comparison point for the tests, I selected one symptom—tingling fingers, or paresthesia—that would provide a point of reference to past, present, and future patients.

J. V. C., a successful dairyman in his fifties, was the first patient who qualified. He had a full range of symptoms, and he felt miserable. After unloading a truck load of hay the day before, he had suffered a pain in his chest and a tingling in his hands and arms. His left arm had cramped. His aches and pains had kept him awake nearly all night.

After administering an electrocardiogram and ruling out coronary thrombosis, I took J. V. C. into my confidence about the B-complex therapy. I explained that I suspected his symptoms might be related to heart disease and that I wanted to see if injected vitamins would help him. It is believed that some patients don't absorb vitamins properly from the intestines. Injection seemed the surest way.

"If it won't kill me and will help science, I'm ready to do it," agreed J. V. C.

In order to have an objective before-and-after record of the therapy I asked my wife, Lucy, a commercial artist whose work illustrates this book, to sketch the patient's hands. Following the QEW test, he flexed the two joints of his fingers as much as he could while Lucy drew his hand exactly as she saw it. He was unable to flex his fingers completely to the palm. There was a space where one could have put a large-sized pencil. Then, beginning that day, he received an arm muscle injection containing 100 milligrams of thiamine, 9.5 milligrams of riboflavin, 150 milligrams of niacinamide, 5 milligrams of panthenol, and 50 milligrams of pyridoxine (B_6). At the end of two weeks Lucy drew his hands again as he flexed them for the QEW test. Now he could flex his fingers completely, pressing the palms with the ends of his fingers. The B-complex injections had done the same as the Morrison diet, pecans, and peanuts had been doing.

One case can mean a lot. It also, for reasons at first unfathomable to the investigator, can sometimes mislead. To make certain I was on the right road, I wanted another patient, this time an active middle-aged woman, on whom to run the experiment a second time.

The patient with the proper specifications came in a few days later. She was fifty-six, big-framed, weighing 190 pounds, and she had tingling hands and couldn't flex her fingers completely. "Every time I sit down to watch television my fingers start tingling and feel numb like they're asleep," she said. "They tingle when

I drive my car to work in the mornings. A lot of times they wake me up in the night tingling. I've sat up half the night lots of times, running warm water over my fingers trying to get some relief." She had chest pain that seemed to spread into her arms and shoulders. Her legs cramped at night. Her fingers were stiff and hurt when she woke up in the mornings. A close look at her hands revealed swollen-looking fingers. They were puffy. She was a perfect patient for the B-complex study, and she was more than willing to participate—anything to get rid of that pain in her chest and fingers.

In order to rule out the possibility of other dietary factors having an effect, I asked her to step up her eating of pork, eggs, butter, and gravies—more animal fats—and we began the series of injections every two days.

Seven injections and two weeks later, she was a remarkably changed woman. "I can see the leaders in my hands better now," she said, and it was certainly true. One could see every tendon on the backs of her hands. The swelling that previously had concealed her tendons was gone. No edema. Although I had given but slight attention to the edema previously, I now realized, as she flexed her fingers perfectly, that it had been edema that had prevented her from flexing them before. This struck me as highly significant. Furthermore, all of her other symptoms had improved. Her chest pain was gone, along with that in her shoulder, arms, and fingers. She hadn't had leg cramps for a week.

And her tingling, my point of comparison, had disappeared.

This indicated, then, that she and the male patient J. V. C. were both deficient in at least one of the five B vitamins I had treated them with. This also seemed to be true of the many others I had placed on the Morrison diet and pecans and peanuts.

This woman's case especially bothered me, for she was a cook in a school cafeteria. She had cooked there for eleven years, each day eating the same selection of food as did the school children and their teachers. My own four children ate every day at the same school cafeteria, a factor that deepened my emotional involvement in my patient's condition. If she got an insufficient supply of B vitamins from the school lunches, the same would be true for the children. This meant a whole generation was embarking on long-term vitamin B deficiencies, sowing the seeds in childhood for future serious medical problems. And if this were happening in one school, might it not also be occurring in other school cafeterias all over the country? I thought so. I also suspected it wasn't only the school cafeterias; it was just as likely to be true of the American eating pattern in general.

It was next necessary to decide which of the B-complex vitamins to test first, and I began pondering the various deficiency symptoms in order to speed up the process of elimination. Three of them seemed to be eliminated automatically. Vitamin B_1 deficiency caused tremors of the tongue; B_2 deficiency, little raw cracks or sores in the corners of the mouth; and nicotinic acid deficiency (the same pellagra that Goldberger had fought), skin lesions of the hands and legs. My patients didn't exhibit any of these three signs. Thus, I ruled out vitamins B_1, B_2, and nicotinic acid. This left two poorly understood vitamins in the injections— B_6 (pyridoxine) and panthenol. Nobody had ever described a syndrome for B_6 deficiency in active adults; I decided to inject vitamin B_6 next. If that didn't work, then panthenol would be tested. If one of those nutrients worked to my satisfaction in improving signs and symptoms, I would thereafter use oral doses of the vitamin, a much preferable and less troublesome method for both physician and patient.

In order to keep the test conditions the same as with the previous patients, it was necessary to obtain a patient of about the same age, with the same symptoms and signs, and consuming the same high-fat diet. I ordered an injectable B_6 preparation, in the form of pyridoxine hydrochloride, and waited for a patient who was markedly suffering from edema—the puffed, swollen condition I had found in the cafeteria cook. Edema was one of the knottiest problems facing medical science. I was convinced, on the basis of my observation of the cook, that one of the vitamins had cleared up her swollen hands. Had it been B_6? I would soon know.

The first patient to receive the vitamin B_6 injection alone was a thirty-seven-year-old Negro woman. She weighed 195 pounds and was eight months pregnant. She had severe tingling in both arms and both hands, and she had swelling in her hands and feet. The tops of her feet were swollen so tightly that her skin had a light sheen to it. It was noticeable from across the room. When I pressed the top of her foot with my finger, the outline of my finger remained several seconds in the swollen flesh of her foot.

"The swelling in my feet has been so bad I had to buy a size larger pair of house shoes," she said. "I couldn't get my regular shoes on and my legs are sore to press on them. When I lie down at night I have cramps in the backs of my legs, between my knees and ankles. Every day after lunch when I get through ironing my clothes and doing my work, I lie down to rest awhile. I no sooner get in bed than the tingling in my hands starts. I feel a numbness up to my elbow."

For my purposes she was a perfect patient, but there were other factors that made me think very carefully about her case. It was May 26, 1962. This meant we were moving into the Texas summer heat, itself trial enough for anybody, much less a woman eight months pregnant. Swelling in the feet and ankles seemed to be more common during the summer months, and this woman had no air conditioning in her home. There was, furthermore, the fact of her being pregnant. Obstetricians had long entertained an old theory that the pressure of the fetus on the veins of the mother's pelvis caused this type of swelling in the feet and legs. Most of them also believed that excessive consumption of table salt caused the swelling, and for years they had advised pregnant women to avoid eating salt. I agreed that Americans ate too much table salt, but now I wasn't sure this was the cause of *edema of pregnancy*. My patient also had symptoms other than swelling. Something else was at work. After consideration of the case and of the patient's individual needs, I went ahead with the B_6 injections, scheduling them 50 milligrams every two days for a two-week period.

Four days later, when she returned for her third injection, what I saw made me hold my breath. I stared at her feet. The skin on top of her feet was as wrinkled as if she had been in swimming too long, and the water had made it pliable and loose. It was an effort for her to keep her feet in the oversize shoes she had bought. Numbness and tingling had left her hands. Puffiness had objectively and dramatically improved in her hands and feet, as had the soreness in her legs. Her right arm still had some residual tingling, but it was obvious that her symptoms were clearing up fast.

In four days, wrinkled, loose skin had replaced tight, puffy hands and feet. She had eaten a diet high in animal fats. There had been no mention of salt. Edema, that big bugaboo of pregnancy, had been reduced by vitamin B₆ alone![16]

It was the greatest thrill I have ever experienced in my medical career.

Rheumatism—As Old as the Greeks | 3

Rheumatism—"any of various painful conditions of the joints and muscles"—goes back at least to the ancient Greeks, who named it, and perhaps even farther. It has been speculated that Neanderthal man of the Paleolithic period was afflicted with it. For the first mention of paresthesia, the medical terms for the numbness and tingling we have already discussed, one goes back at least to Galen, a Greek physician in the second century more than 1,800 years ago. In his early twenties Galen treated gladiators, learning his anatomy from the severely wounded. Later he became court physician to the Roman emperor Marcus Aurelius. One of his patients, who had fallen from a horse, had numbness in the fourth and fifth fingers of one hand. Galen grew intrigued with the belief that nerves came from a central nervous system, and in this patient he reasoned that the numbness had been caused by an injury to the neck vertebrae.[1] However far back in history it may trace, without a doubt rheumatism has brought pain and suffering to millions of persons in many lands.

But what, exactly, is rheumatism? What causes it? What will relieve it? How can it be prevented?

These are large questions, so large that an entire specialty of medicine, rheumatology, is devoted to them. By and large, the questions remain unanswered. This chapter, however, will attempt to answer the questions at least partially.

A precise definition of rheumatism is extremely difficult to arrive at—a problem encountered by the rheumatologist as well as the general practitioner. It has come to be thought of, broadly, as any disease condition of a chronic recurrent nature that involves the connective tissues of the muscles, tendons, bursa, joints, and nerves in the shoulders, arms, hands, hips, legs, neck, and back. In more recent times another term, arthritis, has been vaguely and loosely associated with rheumatism and rheumatismlike conditions.

Although "arthritis" is a commonly used term today by both doctors and patients, I hesitate to use it without very carefully describing what I mean. Arthritis has inspired more controversy, probably, than anything else in medicine. Books purporting to possess the cure for arthritis are numerous, and because of the desperate nature of the persons afflicted with arthritis the books are almost invariably assured a healthy sales. Over the years arthritis has drawn into its orbit more food faddists, steam parlors, masseurs, bath houses, mineral springs, red springs, warm springs, hot springs, charlatans, and just plain quacks than, possibly, any other disease. There have been more patented drugs for arthritis than for almost anything else in medicine. Yet I know of no drugs that significantly help hypertrophic and degenerative arthritis, outside of a few analgesics for pain and adrenocorticotropic hormone. Some doctors have administered a female hormone and claimed some success, but there seems to have been little more than temporary relief.

Rheumatic and arthritic conditions may come from a number of causes, such as bacterial infection, which masks itself as rheumatism. Because these various disease conditions sometimes arise from different causes even though the signs and symptoms are very similar, separating and distinguishing them has been a tedious, laborious task for scientists in different countries, treating different people in different areas. Bacterial infections can cause painful, swollen, and inflamed joints, which is diagnosed as inflammatory arthritis. Rheumatic fever, a condition that may treacherously affect the heart, can also mask itself as rheumatism.

However, the signs and symptoms of the rheumatism I will be

discussing in this chapter are of the idiopathic—or spontan..
and primary—rheumatism that has been a painful experience c
Homo sapiens for centuries. It does not come as the result of a
germ or an injury or a secondary infection. It is, primarily, a
nutritional disease that my patients referred to as "rheumatism."
It was because of the patients with rheumatism that I gained my
earliest and deepest insight into the effectiveness of B_6 therapy.

The range of treatment for rheumatism is amazingly limited.
Before 1961, as many another doctor had done, I treated the disorder with aspirin and buffered aspirin. Once in a while I would
prescribe guarded doses of cortisone, held to a minimum—if the
patient was begging for something to stop pain. Although gold
salts have been used with some success in treatment of rheumatoid
arthritis, buffered aspirin and aspirin therapy is the conventional
method of treatment that is commonly used today.

What I learned about B_6 therapy and rheumatism I learned by
moving gradually from one patient to the next, from one symptom
to another, from one sign to another, slowly and laboriously until
the relationship was obvious. For four years I did very little reading
in the medical literature about rheumatism because I wanted to
have an open mind on the subject. I was trying to see the whole
clinical picture. After I had formed my clinical judgments I could
then read the literature with far more understanding of what the
researchers had found in the laboratory. It was, for me personally,
an experience characterized by a theme of serendipity, of seeking
one thing and happily finding something else, as valuable or
more so.

As I have explained in Chapter 2, the first patient who drew
my attention to these related disease conditions was an oilfield
worker with tingling fingers. All of my work with B_6 eventually
grew from that seminal case. Soon I treated a number of cases of
rheumatism. While questioning patients about diets that seemed
to contain excessive amounts of fat, I learned that numbness and
tingling of the fingers were common symptoms.

This paresthesia of the hands was most noticeable when the
hands were at rest or while the patient was driving an automobile
or lying in bed. When he moved his fingers and rubbed his hands,
the numbness and tingling would subside, only to return later. Oc-

nt would awaken to find an arm temporarily
ould have to rub it or shake it with the other,
to "get the circulation going again." Adults of all
of this. Some of those who seemed worse off
that they had pain in the finger joints when the
xed or "bumped" on objects. The sensitivity was so
even "bumping" the fingers on a bed cover would
bring pain. ...s the symptoms got worse in both men and women,
hand-grip strength began to fail. There seemed to be a failure of
motor power in the hand, somehow, so gradual in its onset that
the patients themselves were not aware of it until, suddenly one
day, they could no longer wring water from a dishcloth or squeeze
milk from a cow's teat. Their disability became more noticeable
at such times, with a corresponding reduction in the speed of finger
movement, especially in flexion and range of flexion.

Invariably I would find numbness, tingling, and loss of sensation
to be in agreement with the anatomical distribution of the digital
nerves arising from the trunk nerves in the arm. Quite frequently,
in early cases, disturbed sensation was limited to the little finger
and the adjacent side of the ring finger. This, for instance, is the
exact terminal distribution of the ulnar nerve in the hand. In other
cases the tingling and numbness would follow the exact distribution
of the median nerve.

The most characteristic sign of this form of rheumatism was the
patient's failure to perform perfectly what I later came to call the
QEW test, described in Chapter 1. Before therapy there was an
obvious disturbance of tendon action, which was caused by swelling
of synovia in the hands. Synovia are thin lining membranes of
bursa, joint cavities, and tendon sheaths. The two finger joints of
the hand could not be flexed completely because of three other
evident factors: impaired nerve, muscle, and tendon motor powers;
swelling of the soft tissues, as well as the joint capsules, of the
fingers; and pain in the finger joints. This, a syndrome known as
"rheumatism," was a condition I was to see over and over through
the years, and it responded to vitamin B_6.

The case history of L. G., a sixty-six-year-old deputy sheriff, is
instructive. On January 20, 1967, he complained, "Doc, I've got
arthritis in my hands, feet, back, and spine." His hands and

fingers were swollen. His legs felt so weakened that he could hardly climb the steps of the county courthouse, a daily routine for a deputy sheriff. For the past two years he had been troubled with a swelling and pain in both knees, and his fingers had been painful longer than that. While driving his automobile he frequently noticed a numbness and tingling in his fingers and hands.

He had been having pains for twenty-four years now, since 1942, the deputy explained to me. His hands and feet had become so swollen that he had been discharged from the Army with a diagnosis of arthritis. From time to time over the years he would improve; then he would have relapses. Now his legs were so stiff and painful that he couldn't cross one leg over the other at the knees while he was sitting. He had been having nocturnal muscle spasms in his legs about two or three nights a week.

A childhood bout with pneumonia had been the extent of his serious illness in the past. Except for the extremities of which he complained, my findings were negative. But there the signs of disease were written large enough for any man to see. His hands and fingers were so swollen that he could barely screw off his ring. Both knees were swollen; there appeared to be a slight amount of fluid in both knee joints. Both feet were marked by slight, diffuse edema. In the interphalangeal joints of his fingers he had lost his flexion by about 50 percent. I gave him 100 milligrams of pyridoxine daily and told him to return in two weeks.

By February 3 the swelling had subsided in the knees, and when he sat down he could cross one leg over the other at the knee—comfortably. He had no pain in the fingers, and his finger flexion, at the interphalangeal joints, was remarkably improved. Numbness and tingling had subsided in the fingers and hands. The swelling in his hands and feet had subsided; now he could more easily remove the ring from his finger.

"I thought I was going to have to retire," he proclaimed happily, "but I can climb the steps of the courthouse without any trouble now."

Three years later, on March 23, 1970, after he had taken pyridoxine (100 milligrams daily) throughout the intervening period, I examined him again. He had no paresthesia of the hands, no swelling in either hands or feet, no swelling in the knees. He did have some tenderness in the finger joints, but it was not to the extent he had had it three years before. His flexion at the inter-phalangeal joints was much better than before treatment back in 1967.

His, it appeared, was a case of the idiopathic, *nutrition-related* rheumatism that has brought agony to millions over the centuries. At his age, 100 milligrams of pyridoxine was used to dispel his symptoms and signs; perhaps at an earlier age half that much would have been sufficient; if he had received an adequate daily supply of pyridoxine as a child—who can say that he would have later suffered his "arthritis"?

There appeared to be a pattern in my patients. As deformity of the finger joints increased, along with disturbed sensation in the fingertips, there eventually was a pronounced impairment of shoulder function and, to some extent, elbows. They commonly complained of pain at both pressure and movement of the shoulders. Yet it was difficult, if not impossible, to determine if the pain about the shoulder came, in a given case, from the synovia of the joint or a nerve or bursa near the joint. In some cases most of the pain was in the arms and was located between the elbows and the shoulders. Simultaneously and insidiously, stiffness tended to develop as the fingers became more deformed. The index finger was affected more than its neighbors. In advanced cases, even when there was little or no edema present, the tip of the index finger could not be made to touch the tip of the thumb. Because of this, housewives became unable to sew, for the thumb and finger could not be approximated enough to use needle and thread. For a woman who was a seamstress by trade or who made some of the family's clothing herself, this presented very serious economic consequences, aside from the pain.

Particularly in women who were near the age of menopause, the finger joints became very painful. Little reddened and exquisitely tender burrs or knots, described by William Heberden in London in 1802 and since called "Heberden's nodes," appeared on the sides of the finger joints. While these also affected the fingers of older men, the condition seemed more attracted to women at or past the age of menopause. Degree of pain and swelling seemed to go together, although some individual joints were more involved than others.

Coordination of finger and hand movement was directly influenced by the degree of impaired flexion. Mechanics dropped screwdrivers, carpenters dropped hammers, and housewives dropped and broke their dishes. Clearly there was, in these instances, an involvement of the nervous system. Patients spoke of the condition as a weakness in the hands; there was a slight tremor and reduced speed when they tried to flex their fingers, and then the fingers were only partially flexed.

Sensation in the fingers was so disturbed in many of the patients that they could not distinguish one substance from another by touch. Housewives could not feel or guide the movements of thimbles on their fingers. Craftsmen often sacrificed employment because of their disabled fingers; they could not meet the requirements for production.

Cramps and muscle spasms were common and were not limited to the hand. In fact, my patients suffered some of their most brutal and forceful muscle spasms in the backs of the legs and arches of the feet, as we saw in the case presented in Chapter 1. Most of the time these cramps occurred at night and were preceded by what was described as a "restless" feeling in the legs. The patients would bolt from their beds in agonizing pain to massage or rub the contracted and knotted muscles in the legs or feet. Aged people sat many nights by their heaters or ran hot water over their feet and legs in efforts to halt the vicious leg cramps.

From time to time a patient was seen—usually a woman near middle age—whose fingers were miserably tight. The skin of the fingers was shiny and glistening white, more so than the rest of the hand, and without wrinkles and quite thin. Frequently she—or he—would grimace, point to the particular finger joint that was the culprit and complain that the joint would lock so that she had to unlock it with the other hand. Some called it a "trigger finger." The patient usually feared that exercising it would set off an involuntary cramp or spasm in the hand or forearm.

Swelling, or edema, usually accompanied the aches and pains. Frequently it was diffuse and barely detectable except by the trained eye. Housewives often complained that their wedding rings had become too tight or that they had to be removed forcibly from their ring fingers. In the more severe cases, the veins and tendons in the backs of their hands were indistinct and the hands appeared "puffy" or "fat."

Younger women experienced an increased amount of swelling in the soft tissues of the hands during the week prior to menstruation. Women frequently told me of discomfort in their hands a day or so before menstruation. In medical circles this has been called "premenstrual edema." Along with it came varying amounts of swelling in the eyelids and the cheeks. Women patients who already had finger and joint pain usually had increased finger and joint pain during the day or so before menstruation.

Because of a possible relationship between it and the elastic connective tissue in the body, one more sign should be described. Some patients suffering from a long-standing rheumatic disease in the hands had no wrinkles there. This held true even in some of the aged. Instead, in the cheek of the face there was this same glistening, shiny sheen that characterized the skin of the tight, stiffened, and almost fixed fingers. The relationship here between edema and the connective tissue of both hands and face is of particular interest to us. Histologists long ago demonstrated that the cheeks of the face, not the whole face, are composed of cells that contain a remarkably high percentage of elastic connective tissues. It seems probable that the same mechanism that made the hands tight and glistening also was at work in the tissues of the face—and perhaps elsewhere, as we will see in subsequent chapters.

In dealing with these various conditions that can be lumped generally under the diagnosis of "rheumatism," after a few months of clinical study I began prescribing oral doses of pyridoxine. Usually 50 milligrams were given daily, and all the symptoms I have listed here responded to the therapy. Pain was relieved or eradicated. Function was restored. After a period of time I was able to establish a timetable for improvement or recession of symptoms. Some patients experienced a return to health within a week or two; some, in six weeks; others, usually the elderly, had gradual improvement, up to six and eight months.

Hand grip, for instance, was usually restored dramatically. One well-dressed woman with expensive rings could not touch the tips of her fingers to her palm when she first came in. After eight days of B_6 therapy she could do this exercise with facility. Disabled dairymen, who could no longer squeeze the teats of a cow, took 50 milligrams of B_6 and by the end of two weeks were milking, by hand, a half-dozen cows a day. These cases undoubtedly also involved an improvement in motor-nerve physiology, related to the reduction of swelling at the wrist. Let us examine in detail the case of L. C. S., aged fifty-six.

L. C. S. had been a successful dairyman for twenty-five years and a swine grower for the past five years when I first observed him on March 15, 1966. His signs and symptoms were numerous. They included, in the sometimes technical medical language that I used on his chart, bilateral numbness and tingling in the fingers and hands; swelling of fingers and hands; "trigger finger" of right ring finger of the right hand; failure to flex tips of the fingers to touch metacarpophalangeal crease in either palm (QEW test); painful interphalangeal finger joints; weakness of hand grip in his right hand; painful elbows; periarticular swelling around both knees; occasional nocturnal paralysis of the entire left arm such that, on awakening, the unaffected hand would be used to massage and shake the affected arm and hand to return of function; and point tenderness near the tips of the acromion (the outer extremity of the shoulder) in both shoulders.

He had been assaulted, it seemed, by a plague of painful, abnormal conditions, whether one called them arthritis or "just plain ol' rheumatism." Although each of the signs and symptoms was enough to cause complaint, his finger joints were quite painful even when they were only passively squeezed or massaged. In most cases this could be used as a general index of the severity of a patient's condition.

Treatment began with daily oral doses of 50 milligrams of pyridoxine, with no discussion of diet. No other medication was prescribed.

On April 4, three weeks later, L. C. S. reported an overall general improvement. An increased wrinkling of the skin on the hands and fingers indicated a reduction in edema. He passed the QEW test by flexing *all* his fingers to touch the metacarpophalangeal crease of each palm. His right hand grip had returned to normal, and the numbness and tingling in his hands and fingers had subsided. The nocturnal paralysis of his left arm had been relieved. The "trigger finger" problem in his right ring finger had disappeared. The pain in his shoulders was improved but not completely relieved. The pain in his knees, as well as the periarticular swelling of the knees, had lessened. In all, he had enjoyed about as much improvement as a doctor is likely to hope for in such a short period of time.

The photographs in this chapter give a before-and-after photographic record of L. C. S.'s medical experience. Although the

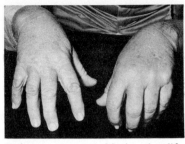 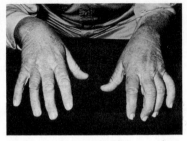

Before treatment—Notice the diffuse swelling (edema) in the hands and fingers.

After treatment—After patient had taken 50 milligrams of pyridoxine daily for 21 days, there was a noticeable reduction of swelling (edema) in the hands and fingers.

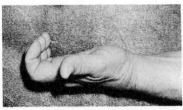 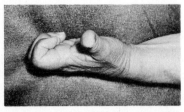

Before treatment—Notice that with the wrist and hand extended, the fingers could not be flexed at the interphalangeal joints.

After treatment—Having taken 50 milligrams of pyridoxine daily for 21 days, patient could flex his fingers at the interphalangeal joints.

A Dairyman's Hands (Figs. 3–6)

pictures depict graphically how much better L. C. S. could flex and manipulate his hands after treatment with pyridoxine, it is perhaps even more impressive that before he had completed the first three weeks of therapy he had already begun milking several cows a day again!

Six weeks after initial therapy with pyridoxine had begun, the pain and swelling had subsided around all joints except that of the right knee. There, the swelling was less, but pain continued, although there was considerably less than before treatment.

In an informal follow-up examination six years later, on April 24, 1972, I saw L. C. S. at a cattlemen's meeting. During that six-year period he had taken 50 milligrams of pyridoxine daily. Still actively employed in livestock production, he had better use of his shoulders, arms, and hands than when the photographs were made. He had no edema in his hands, and he could flex his fingers perfectly.

L. C. S.'s case is not an isolated one. I have seen patients, time and time again, who could not pull open the front door of my office because of the excruciating pain in their fingers. Within three weeks a daily dosage of B_6 would enable them to open the door by themselves. Most frequently these patients were of middle age. There is something about middle-aged persons that is different, probably a hormone imbalance or deficiency in both men and women, and it responds to pyridoxine.

It seems likely that the pain in the fingers is caused by actual degeneration, or melting away, so to speak, of the coverings of the little nerves that go to the nerves—the myelin sheaths. It has been proved that dogs subjected to B_6 deficiency actually develop a sloughing or degeneration of myelin sheaths of the sciatic nerves in the backs of their legs. This indicates, as do the reported signs and symptoms, that patients with painful fingers have a nerve, as well as bone, disease. Tingling is the first signal that B_6 is needed; pain develops later, followed by edema and stiffness of the joints. In association with it there is both swelling and deformity of the joints, and this is usually diagnosed as osteoarthritis.

The very earliest stages of a disease or deficiency condition are rarely seen in a physician's office. Invariably the patient will not bother with a medical problem until it reaches the point where it gives him more than a little concern. In many instances the patient does not go to the doctor until the condition has become either too painful to abide or of significant economic consequence to him.

The case of N. S., fifty-three, first seen on July 1, 1966, illustrates my point. N. S., a janitor in a barbershop who also shined shoes, came in because his means of earning a living was in jeopardy.

"My fingers and hands go to sleep night and day, and my hand grip has gone," he said. He could no longer clutch a rag with enough strength to shine shoes. His hands and fingers continuously tingled with a "pins-and-needles" sensation, as if he had been "lying on the hands too long." The plight of his fingers, now very painful, had been getting steadily worse for several years. For the same period of time he had been gradually developing a stiffness in his fingers.

For the past year or more he had suffered with very severe nocturnal muscle spasms in his legs that forced him out of bed at night to massage the cramps from his legs. Every other night, on the average, he was awakened by these painful muscle spasms, which he called "cally hawks," apparently a classification of his own invention. But he had suffered through it all until he was no longer able to shine shoes. His joints hurt when he pulled on the shine rag, which, now that he was too weak to grip it, would drop from his hands.

In his medical history it was noted that about two years before he had noticed some loss of facial expression, which had been diagnosed as early Parkinson's disease.

As for positive findings in his physical, his face was rather expressionless, in keeping with Parkinson's disease, and there was a glistening sheen in the cheeks, indicating swelling there. In his extremities he had a diffuse swelling of the hands and fingers, and the dorsum of the hands was especially puffy in appearance. Going through the QEW test with difficulty, he displayed a marked reduction in his ability to flex his fingers at the interphalangeal joints. There was, as well, impaired coordination of finger movements and stiffness in the finger joints. His hand grip was considerably poorer than that which would be expected in a man of his age and size.

Pyridoxine (50 milligrams daily by mouth) was prescribed, and as was true with other cases presented, and to be presented, in this book (unless otherwise stipulated), diet was not altered and food was not discussed. My reason for not changing anything else in his, and others', routine was to make absolutely certain that B_6 alone was responsible for the improvements noted. Therefore, it was the only variable in this and other cases.

N. S. returned to the office six weeks later, on August 15. The skin was wrinkled on the skin of the dorsum of both hands; even without this evidence it was clear that his hands and fingers were less swollen. He reported that the tingling pins-and-needles paresthesia had subsided in both fingers and hands, the brutally painful nocturnal spasms or "cally hawks" had subsided, the finger joints were no longer painful, and his hand grip had improved enough that he could clutch his rag and shine shoes. His range of finger flexion was improved some, but he was by no means completely improved in this respect, for there remained residual stiffness at the interphalangeal joints. But, most importantly, *N. S. was back in business and could make a living.*

He continued on B_6 (50 milligrams daily) for three years. When I saw him on March 4, 1969, he had no complaints about his hands except residual stiffness. There had been no recurrence of paresthesia in the hands and no difficulty with nocturnal spasms or cramps in the muscles of the legs. His hand grip continued to be strong, and he seemed as able, and as willing, to work as ever.

"I can pop that shine rag now like I want to!" he declared.

While the outlook is optimistic for most rheumatism sufferers treated with B_6, as we have seen in the foregoing cases and photographs, I hasten to emphasize that two disorders of the joints have not responded to B_6, in my experience: traumatic arthritis, caused by injury, and rheumatoid arthritis. For purposes of distinction I prefer to set traumatic arthritis (due to injury) to one side, and then to divide the remaining cases into rheumatism and rheumatoid arthritis. Rheumatoid arthritis has a different etiology that is unrelated to B_6.

In my experience clear-cut and distinctive rheumatoid arthritis did not respond to vitamin B_6. Interestingly enough, however, some relationship seems to have been established between rheumatoid-arthritis patients and B_6 deficiency by other investigators. Patients with this disorder did excrete increased amounts of xanthurenic acid and kynurenine, two of the abnormal metabolites of the amino-acid tryptophan, which would indicate an increased need for pyridoxine in order to handle tryptophan properly. This is one of the puzzling aspects of this particular form of arthritis. Dr. H. Spiera, chief of the Arthritis Clinic at Mt. Sinai Hospital in New York, stated: "It is impossible to assess the significance of the abnormal excretion of tryptophan metabolites by patients with rheumatoid arthritis. It does not seem to be related to tissue destruction, pyridoxine deficiency, inflammation, gamma globulin turnover, or to drugs used in the management of rheumatoid arthritis."[2] But, adds Dr. Spiera, because nothing is known of the etiology or pathogenesis of rheumatoid arthritis, any differences such as the increased xanthurenic-acid excretions should be explored.

Isobel M. Bett of the Rheumatic Diseases Unit of the Northern General Hospital in Edinburgh has noted that pyridoxine restores normal metabolism of patients who had excreted elevated metabolites. Nonetheless, as in the experience of others, excretion of these metabolites did not correlate well with the disease's clinical activity. In one series of clinical studies, Bett reported results that tended to support earlier investigators who suggested that low urinary pyridoxine did not necessarily mean low availability in the body and that it could be used up at an unusually rapid rate in these patients by some other metabolic or immunological process. Bett thought that any pyridoxine deficiency in patients with rheumatoid arthritis was probably a relatively mild one. However, there were other puzzling sides to the whole question. "Patients whose tryptophan metabolism became normal on pyridoxine did not necessarily improve clinically," wrote Bett. "On the other hand, in those who did improve, kynurenine excretion tended to fall."[3] Kynurenine is another metabolite of tryptophan, the high excretion of which indicates a pyridoxine need.

In an earlier study, Bett had reported that prolonged administration of pyridoxine to patients who had rheumatoid arthritis had brought about a fall in kynurenine in tryptophan-load tests. When pyridoxine was withdrawn, kynurenine was again excreted in increased amounts. These results occurred in a majority of patients.[4]

Before that, in 1961, investigators A. B. McKusick and J. M. Hsu had reported a syndrome similar to the shoulder-hand syndrome of rheumatoid arthritis in patients with tuberculosis who were being treated with the drug isoniazid and PAS, or para-amino-salicylic acid. When the drug was removed, or else was accompanied by pyridoxine, the patient improved.[5] It should be noted that pyridoxine had earlier been used in tubercular patients as a means of counteracting some side effects of the drug isoniazid.

Parents of children with rheumatoid arthritis have asked me if B_6 might help them. I have explained very carefully that I recommend, with children having rheumatoid arthritis, that they be given 25 milligrams of B_6 morning and night, *with the expectation that the signs and symptoms will not change unless they also have these other signs and symptoms that are not necessarily associated with rheumatoid arthritis.* In other words, B_6 can do no harm, but by the same token it may do no good either, unless the patient also has one of the other conditions that I have earlier described as "rheumatism." I have had patients who had two different conditions—rheumatoid arthritis, which did not change, and rheumatism, which did change when B_6 was given.

Despite the fact that B_6 has not achieved clinical success with rheumatoid arthritis, it must be remembered that laboratory data based on the tryptophan-load test and subsequent excretion of kynurenine and xanthurenic acid indicate that B_6 is needed by the majority of those patients suffering from rheumatoid arthritis.

Because the objective findings in the hands of these patients I successfully treated for rheumatism were so apparent to patients and doctors alike, I would like to outline briefly the results obtained by pyridoxine. The ten main features include:

1. Reduced edema
2. Reduced pain
3. Improved range of flexion
4. Increased speed of flexion
5. Eliminated locking of finger joints
6. Increased strength of grip
7. Improved sensation

8. Improved coordination
9. Reduced stiffness
10. Sustained flexion

These changes in the hands could usually be related to improvement elsewhere in the body. Reduction of edema, for example, invariably occurred over the rest of the body as well as the hands. Almost without fail, hitherto tight wedding rings became looser; many women feared they would lose their rings down the kitchen drain pipe. On the average there was a weight loss from five to seven pounds following pyridoxine treatment. The reduction of edema was also evident in other ways. Before treatment, a patient's cheeks often were shiny, almost glistening, and devoid of wrinkles, just as the fingers were tight and shiny. After pyridoxine, the skin in both the hands and the cheeks gradually relaxed, in time forming tiny wrinkles and losing the characteristic shiny skin coloring.

Although it was found in only a few cases, the cold perspiration of the palms indicated a severe abnormality in some patients. Paroxysms of palm sweating would appear for a few minutes and then wane. This was most likely caused by pressure of swollen synovia on the median nerve. The patients had cold, moist fingers at normal room temperature. After pyridoxine, the fingers became warm and dry and remained so.

Pain is an experience difficult to gauge and difficult to trace. Obviously the patient is the best judge of where and how a portion of his body hurts. It is simple for him to determine *if* he has pain, but it is not always so simple to pinpoint precisely where the pain is or how it may have come about. He is certain, however, when the pain appears—and when it disappears. Painful interphalangeal joints, common among my patients, were relieved to some extent within three weeks of beginning treatment. Most were substantially improved at the end of six weeks. Elderly patients who already had deformity of their fingers improved gradually for months and even years. In hands where there was no deformity to begin with, pain was relieved in the fingers more completely, in both men and women. Heberden's nodes, the painful little burrs or knots, became less painful and, in some instances, smaller.

Shoulder pain was an important symptom in patients who had

severe pathological changes in their hands. However, it was quite hard to locate exactly where the pain stemmed from, because the nerves, bursa, and capsule of the shoulder joints are in such close proximity. Yet this shoulder pain—to be distinguished from traumatic bursitis, which would not respond—responded to pyridoxine. Elbow pain also had a vague, indistinct location, making it difficult to determine if the pain was in the synovia or nerves or both. I entertained suspicion that it came from the synovia. Pyridoxine relieved elbow pain in about six weeks. Hip pain seemed to be in the hip joint, and to some extent it responded to pyridoxine. Knee pain, even more difficult to evaluate, showed some response to pyridoxine. A few patients showed reduction of swelling in the area of the knees within two weeks; as swelling subsided, knee pain improved.

Paresthesia—numbness and tingling—was the most frequently mentioned symptom that was treated with B_6, and it was the one most successfully relieved. When 50 milligrams of pyridoxine were given daily, paresthesia was relieved within two weeks. Nocturnal paralysis of an arm was relieved completely within two weeks, and nocturnal muscle cramps, a very common complaint with patients who had pathological changes in their hands, were usually relieved within one week.

Hand grip was restored within two weeks and often dramatically in less time. By some unexplained means there was a restoration of motor power, probably as a result of improved motor-nerve physiology.

Definite improvement of sensation in the fingertips usually came within two weeks. As paresthesia got better, so did sensation. Patients previously unable to feel the weave of cloth could do so after treatment; a seamstress then could close her eyes and distinguish what type of cloth was between her fingers merely by touch.

Improved sensation, speed of flexion, and range of flexion seemed to lead to better coordination of finger movements. Mechanics and carpenters no longer dropped their screwdrivers and hammers; housewives held on to their teacups and dishes; elderly women resumed sewing with thimble, needle, and thread. Finger stiffness was improved within six weeks, with the fingers becoming more pliable. This also seemed to accompany other, generalized improvement. For example, elderly women could get in and out of bed or the bathtub easier than before. There was more power and strength in their legs.

A key to success in treatment was the index finger. The index finger was the stiffest, most difficult finger of all to improve. It was the last finger that could be made to flex completely. The reason for this lies in the fact that the anatomy of the index finger is remarkable in its difference from its three neighbors. The muscle bellies of the flexor digitorum profundus tendons that insert into the little, ring, and long fingers of the hand are all grouped in a common muscle sheath, and motor power is supplied by the ulnar nerve. But the flexor digitorum profundus of the index finger is separate; it is supplied by the median nerve for motor power, and the median nerve also supplies sensation for the index finger. Spontaneous compression of the median nerve at the carpal tunnel is probably the reason why the index finger is stiffer than the other fingers. Also, this anatomical difference explains the longer wait for the index finger to improve. Motion pictures I took of several patients, before treatment and six weeks afterward, clearly revealed that improvement in the flexion of the index finger was slower and required a longer period of therapy than did the others. Index fingers normally required six weeks of therapy before improving.

Exercise seemed to make symptoms and signs worse. For instance, after twelve or fourteen days of treatment with pyridoxine, a patient's finger pain and swelling would substantially subside. Yet if the fingers were repeatedly flexed, after a night of rest, within minutes one or two of the affected fingers would become swollen and painful. After pyridoxine had been used long enough, exercise failed to cause this discomfort.

It is a simple solution to a medical problem that has plagued patients for ages; yet it has proved itself to be effective and without harmful side effects. This is what the patient hopes for and needs.

The ancient Greeks—and Neanderthal man, no doubt—would have called it miraculous.

Rheumatism and the Carpal Tunnel Syndrome | 4

As I worked more and more with vitamin B₆ therapy, it became apparent that many of the signs and symptoms I had assembled by then coincided almost perfectly with those known to the orthopedic surgeons as the carpal tunnel syndrome.

The carpal tunnel (from the medical term *carpus*, meaning wrist) is a small compartment in the hand enclosed by bone and covered by dense ligament. For twenty-five years the carpal tunnel has been explored and described meticulously by orthopedic surgeons in many university centers. Through this carpal tunnel pass flexor tendons that go to the fingers, synovia (a thin slick sheath that covers the tendons), and the median nerve (a thick nerve the size of a kitchen match). As they removed the overlying ligament, the surgeons have studied the synovia, the nerve, and the tendons in great detail.

The carpal tunnel syndrome, roughly, includes all conditions that produce irritation or compression of the median nerve within the carpal tunnel. As has been pointed out by one investigator, George S. Phalen, M.D.,* for twenty-five years a surgeon at Cleveland Clinic and an authority in the field, "The majority of patients

* Now of the Dallas Medical and Surgical Clinic.

with the carpal-tunnel syndrome give no history of injury to their wrists before the onset of the symptoms."[1]

Diagnosis of the syndrome is based on three major clinical signs: hypesthesia, or impaired feeling; Tinel's sign, a tingling sensation that radiates out into the hand; and a positive wrist-flexion test. Phalen described the wrist-flexion test in the *Journal of the American Medical Association* in 1951. This test consists of holding the wrist in complete flexion for a period of from thirty to sixty seconds. As the wrist is flexed, the median nerve is squeezed between ligament and tendons. If the syndrome is present, this almost immediately worsens the numbness and paresthesia in the fingers.

The layman may be a bit confused by the seeming technicality of differentiating carpal tunnel syndrome from rheumatism and may think this distinction sounds like nit-picking or a sudden, unexpected sprint into a jungle of medical jargon. But actually, as we will see, the carpal tunnel syndrome is one that links every one of the major disorders discussed in this book.

This also inspires a series of questions: What is arthritis? What is rheumatism? Bursitis? Neuritis? Synovitis? These questions cover the whole field of rheumatology. There are volumes and volumes written on it. Unfortunately, a clear-cut differentiation of these conditions is difficult. When one is dealing with acroparesthesia, carpal tunnel syndrome, menopausal arthritis (particularly the swelling of Heberden's nodes), and diffuse edema that respond to pyridoxine, there is not going to be a clear-cut name applied to them all. These conditions have been vague, ill-defined, and, until now, misunderstood.

I have given a prominent position in this chapter to the carpal tunnel syndrome because of the attention the medical literature has been giving it in relatively recent years. For nearly a century now the literature has discussed paresthesia of the hands. During more recent times the orthopedic surgeons have shown that much of this paresthesia of the hands was a spontaneous compression of the median nerve.

It has further been my own clinical experience that many of these hands have diffuse edema on the back as well as the volar surface, or palm. This edema, of course, may arise separately and apart from the true carpal tunnel syndrome. But a trained eye can see this edema throughout the arm and the face, and if one looks down at the feet and ankles one will often see edema there, too.

One of the most significant features of the carpal tunnel syndrome is that Phalen and a number of others have associated the carpal tunnel syndrome with a heretofore undiagnosed systemic disease. Also, as we will see in this chapter, the carpal tunnel syndrome is inseparably associated with a hormone and B$_6$ relationship. The carpal tunnel syndrome appears during pregnancy, with the use of the birth-control pill, and more frequently in persons who have a family history of diabetes.

These are significant distinctions. In the past, certainly in the minds of many patients and other non-doctors, rheumatism has been thought popularly to be conditions of the joints and muscles. Although in Chapter 3 we have shown some links between rheumatism and the nerves, the carpal tunnel syndrome ties the nerves in even closer to rheumatism, while additionally implicating the hormones.

In the medical literature, the carpal tunnel syndrome is inseparably associated with *acroparesthesia*, a tingling and numbness, coldness and pallor of the hands. Dr. James Jackson Putnam, a Harvard Medical School professor writing in the *Archives of Medicine* in 1880, described virtually all of these symptoms that have intrigued me—namely, the numbness and tingling paresthesias of the hands. Putnam's work with the nervous system is of more than passing interest to us here. He was one of the important pioneers of both structural and functional neurology and a founder of the American Neurological Association in 1875 and later its president. In 1872 Dr. Putnam established one of the first neurological clinics in the United States, at Massachusetts General Hospital, and he continued to work there until 1909. He taught at Harvard from 1872 to 1912. Putnam's neurological interests also led him into an association with Sigmund Freud, the father of psychoanalysis. Putnam published the first paper in English that was specifically on psychoanalysis; he later became an early defender and friend of Freud.[2] Over the years the two men maintained an active correspondence.[3]

These paresthesias of the hands, then, were described as long ago as 1880, and at that time they were thought related to neurology rather than to surgery. Since then different medical literature of the world has presented evidence on acroparesthesia. Acroparesthesia and the carpal tunnel syndrome are inseparably associated. The carpal tunnel syndrome is apparently an advanced degree of acroparesthesia, with swelling of the synovia that press on the median nerve in the carpal tunnel. In rheumatism, there is an associated pain in the elbow and pain in the shoulder, which some authorities relate with carpal tunnel syndrome, and the patient with acroparesthesia almost invariably has vague and ill-defined pain in the shoulders and arms. These symptoms definitely connect carpal tunnel syndrome with rheumatism.

Phalen has pointed out that more women than men suffer from the carpal tunnel syndrome. In a 1970 article in the *Journal of the American Medical Association*, dealing with data from 379 patients and involving 597 hands, Phalen established the ratio of women to men as three to one. "Since the majority of patients with carpal tunnel syndrome are women at or near the menopause, hormonal changes may be playing some causative role," he concluded.[4] The cause of the swelling and of the compression of the median nerve had never been determined, as far as I have been able to determine, until my own investigations led to the use of B_6 therapy. B_6 therapy has proved to be successful in patients suffering from this syndrome, described by Phalen as "by far the most common single cause of pain, numbness, and tingling in the hands at night." Objective response, recorded in motion pictures of my patients, has been registered within four to six weeks after the first pyridoxine tablets were taken, with hand function improved, along with a reduction of pain in the arms, elbows, and shoulders, which was, in effect, rheumatism.

Although description of the syndrome has evolved over a period of nearly a hundred years, the carpal tunnel syndrome was first listed as a disease entity by the *Index Medicus* in 1965. Since it is a sign-and-symptom complex resulting from tropic, motor, and sensory changes caused by pressure on the median nerve as it courses through the carpal tunnel, the disease complex may involve one or both hands.

A brief recapitulation of the syndrome's origins in the medical literature takes one back to Putnam's description in 1880 of intense numbness of the hands from the wrist down, which was apart from Raynaud's disease (a syndrome of vascular spasm and deterioration in digital arteries), and a similar description of paresthesia of the hand that was named "acroparesthesia" by the German, F. Schultze, in 1893. Many investigators in both Europe and the United States have listed various causes of pressure on the median nerve at the carpal tunnel. These include fractures of the radius and other trauma at the wrist, infections, ganglions (small tumors growing on tendons), calcific tendonitis (inflamed, calcified tendon), pregnancy, and a number of systemic diseases.[5] (See Fig. 7.)

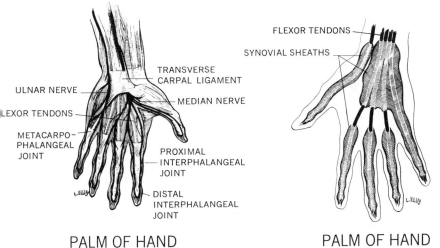

FLEXOR TENDONS

SYNOVIAL SHEATHS

TRANSVERSE CARPAL LIGAMENT

ULNAR NERVE

MEDIAN NERVE

LEXOR TENDONS

METACARPO-PHALANGEAL JOINT

PROXIMAL INTERPHALANGEAL JOINT

DISTAL INTERPHALANGEAL JOINT

PALM OF HAND

PALM OF HAND

Fig. 7. Drawings of the carpal tunnel

Drs. B. W. Cannon and J. G. Love in 1946 first reported sectioning the transverse carpal ligament (as shown in drawing) to relieve pressure on the median nerve,[6] and a year later W. R. Brain, A. D. Wright, and M. Wilkinson reported surgical treatment of six cases of spontaneous compression of the median nerve by sectioning the transverse carpal ligament.[7] As it evolved, this was surgical treatment of the carpal tunnel syndrome.

Subsequently Phalen, in a 439-patient series beginning in 1947, gave monumental descriptions of the syndrome and provided enlightenment on the pathogenesis within the carpal tunnel. He found the synovia covering the flexor tendons of the fingers to be thickened and edematous in many instances. During biopsies of the synovia, histologic, or cellular, examination revealed fibrosis in eighty specimens, chronic inflammation in forty-six, and no change in twenty-two. Weaknesses of varying degrees were found in 41 percent of the hands, and this was attributed to atrophy of the median nerve supplying the opponens pollicis, abductor pollicis brevis, and flexor pollicis brevis muscles. These are the muscles of the hand that draw the thumb to touch the other fingers.

Phalen pointed out that 27.2 percent of the patients in his series either had diabetes or had a history of diabetes in their families— a significant association. Other systemic disorders that indicated hormone imbalance included myxedema (a constitutional disorder due to a decrease or absence of thyroid hormone, characterized by a sallow, puffy appearance, especially of the face and hands) and acromegaly (a disease in which there is permanent enlargement of the bones of the head, hands, and feet, caused by abnormal activity of the pituitary gland). Other frequently found disease conditions included "trigger finger" or "trigger thumb," rheumatoid arthritis, periarthritis of the shoulder, and "tennis elbow."[8]

After treating hundreds of my own patients with pyridoxine for paresthesia and edema of the hands, it eventually occurred to me, after reading the reports of Phalen and others, that signs and symptoms of many of my patients coincided with those of "acroparesthesia," "carpal tunnel syndrome," and "shoulder-hand syndrome." During the preceding years I had learned that pyridoxine would relieve premenstrual edema, the edema of pregnancy, menopausal arthritis, and the edema associated with the use of antiovulatory hormones, all of which was published in an autobiographical account in 1966.[9] And what made the carpal tunnel syndrome of greatest interest was that it moved the concepts of paresthesia away from the circulatory system and redirected medical thought toward the contents of the carpal tunnel: tendons, synovia, and the median nerve, none of which had any direct association with the arterial and venous circulation of the hand. This was something new, indeed, and the changed thought it produced would necessarily have an impact on the medical views of disorders in other parts of the body.

During the ten-year period from 1962 to 1972 I administered pyridoxine (50–1,000 milligrams daily) to about 225 pregnant women, depending on the amount of edema in their hands and feet. There were a number of expectant mothers who had all the criteria necessary for a diagnosis of the carpal tunnel syndrome. As we will see in Chapter 7, these pregnant women experienced relief from nocturnal paresthesia identified as numbness and tingling in the fingers and hands, weakness of hand grip, inadvertent dropping of objects, incoordination of finger movements, and swelling in hands and fingers. Most significantly, tactile sensation was restored in the fingertips that were supplied by the median nerve, definitely tying in the hormones and the nerves to this syndrome.

As an objective sign to indicate improvement, I used the QEW test with my patients before and after treatment. Before treatment with pyridoxine there was often an incomplete flexion of the fingers at the proximal and distal interphalangeal joints. After therapy, flexion was improved and the patient could perform the QEW test satisfactorily.

After achieving this initial success with pregnant patients I observed similar response with the same signs and symptoms in non-pregnant patients, which otherwise would have been diagnosed as rheumatism or some variation of periarthritis and arthritis. Here, too, the QEW test was used to measure the effects of pyridoxine.

Again, pyridoxine would restore maximum finger flexion—provided the rheumatism and periarthritis had not existed for too many years. Unlike the pregnant patients, in the second group I was dealing also with older persons who might have suffered for a number of years before taking pyridoxine. Usually, however, age did not hamper the beneficial effects of B_6.

Two case histories will identify the carpal tunnel syndrome and demonstrate its response to pyridoxine.

Case 1: L. S., thirty-three, a clerk-typist, first observed on November 27, 1971, complained that ten days previously her right hand had become so "weak" that if she tried to pick up an object she would drop it. The hand felt "asleep" or numb. She had difficulty holding a pencil and had to use her index and long fingers because of a disabled thumb. She reported finger spasms, necessitating their massage. For the past month her right hand would wake her at night; she got relief by hanging it over the side of the bed. At times her fingers swelled, making her birthstone ring tight. Her thumb felt weak and its joint felt as if it was "out of place" when she moved the thumb. She had no problem with her left hand.

For the past ten years L. S. had been taking an antiovulatory contraceptive pill, except for cyclic omission three days before each menstruation. For the past six years she had taken no vitamin supplements of any type.

During examination she exhibited pain when I pressed the volar (palm) surface of the wrist of her right hand, and the pain radiated up the volar surface of the arm for 10 centimeters. Comparing the right with the left hand, I perceived a slight edema that was not present in the left. There was also a cold perspiration on the palm and weakness in the abductor muscles of the right thumb.

Her lab results showed a normal uric acid level of 2.9 milligrams percent, urine negative for sugar and albumin, a blood count of 21,600 white blood cells with 81 percent polymorphs, and a quite high hemoglobin level of 14.4 grams. Thus, laboratory tests were negative of disease clues.

While still in the office I gave her a single c.c. of B-complex vitamins, injected intravenously. The injection contained 50 milligrams of pyridoxine, and she was instructed to take 50 milligrams orally, night and morning, and to resume work.

Three days later, on November 30, she experienced reduction of the edema. Her ring could be removed easily, and the numbness and tingling in the thumb, index, long, and ring fingers had completely subsided. All pain in the hand and in the lower volar portion of the forearm had also completely subsided. The only sign that remained was the cold perspiration of her palm.

Four days after that—on December 4, one full week after starting pyridoxine—she remained asymptomatic and noted that she was now able to lift a skillet as easily as she ever had. For a month and a half before therapy, she said, she hadn't been able to grip a skillet handle strongly enough to take the skillet off the stove.

Four weeks after her first visit—on December 24—a careful examination of her hand revealed residual weakness of the thenar muscles of the right hand, which were smaller and softer than those of left hand. Her thumb movement was improved in coordination, and she had no pain at the metacarpophalangeal joint of the thumb. Although the cold perspiration of the right palm was definitely improved, it still continued to a slight degree.

By January 19, 1972, L. S. had no pain, paresthesia, or swelling in the right hand, and I discharged her with instructions to continue taking 50 milligrams morning and night.

During all this time she had continued in her job as clerk-typist. Of her own choosing, she continued taking the contraceptive anti-ovulatory pill.

Case 2: A. F., twenty-one, appeared in my office on June 1, 1967, with edema in her hands and feet. She had had a positive pregnancy test in May; her last menstrual period had been March 13, 1967. She weighed 192 pounds. On her first office visit I prescribed a prenatal vitamin-mineral capsule containing 10 milligrams of pyridoxine, along with an additional 50 milligrams of pyridoxine, providing her a daily total of 60 milligrams.

One month later, on July 1, the edema had subsided completely. But by August 1 the swelling had recurred. Her wedding rings were tight. So were her shoes. Her feet and legs exhibited a pitting edema. At this point I increased pyridoxine to a total daily intake of 110 milligrams. Within one week the edema had totally subsided.

It began to appear as if we were playing a game of oneupmanship with edema, for by October 1 the swelling returned. This time pyridoxine was increased to 160 milligrams daily, again routing the edema. Then on November 17 she again turned up with a pitting edema of the feet and legs and an obvious swelling of the fingers and hands. She complained of her fingers feeling tight and of pain when she moved the joints of her fingers. She could not execute the QEW test. Pyridoxine was duly increased, this time to 310 milligrams a day, and on November 24—seven days later —there were tiny wrinkles on the dorsum of both feet, the skin on her hands was loose, the pain in her finger joints had subsided, and all her fingers could be flexed efficiently in the QEW test.

During the last thirty days of her pregnancy she received 310 milligrams of pyridoxine daily. She was admitted to the hospital in labor on December 19 with no edema in the hands and no pitting edema of the ankles. Her weight gain had been eighteen pounds during the period, and her blood pressure was 170/110 mm. mercury. The fetus was in a breech position, and because of this, following spontaneous labor on that date, I performed a Caesarean-section delivery without complication for either mother or infant.

In A. F.'s family history she had a brother who was mentally retarded to a great extent (he was not a Mongoloid), and her paternal grandfather had died with diabetes as his main complication. In 1968, the year after I had delivered A. F.'s baby, A. F.'s paternal aunt, then sixty-seven, developed acroparesthesia of the hands, and her hands became so painful that she could not grip a well rope sufficiently to draw a bucket of water, as was necessary on the farm where she lived. Nor could she raise her arms because of the pain in her shoulders. The condition had reached the stage that all of her dresses had to be made specially so that she could step into them, obviating the necessity of slipping them on over-head, because she couldn't raise her arms and hands over her head. Apparently referred to me by A. F., the aunt was given 50 milligrams of pyridoxine daily. I examined this patient several times during the next eight months, and after eight months of therapy the acroparesthesia of the hands had subsided, her shoulders were no longer painful, she could draw water from the well easily, and she could slip a dress over her head with her arms raised. Not only was this remarkable to her, but on January 15, 1972, after four years of continuing pyridoxine supplements (50 milligrams daily), she remained free of pain in her shoulders, arms, and hands.

As for A. F., the original patient, three years following the Caesarean delivery she developed severe pain in the right hand, arm, and shoulder. At this time, December 15, 1970, she was not pregnant, but as previously her right hand was swollen and ex-hibited weakness, her fingers would not flex completely for the QEW test, and she couldn't write with a pencil. Her symptoms qualified for a diagnosis of carpal tunnel syndrome.

She was given 50 milligrams of pyridoxine three times a day for a total of 150 milligrams. In three days the pain had completely subsided in the right hand, arm, and shoulder; swelling had subsided in the hand and fingers; hand function had returned to normal.

It would be difficult for me to enumerate how many patients with aspects of the carpal tunnel syndrome were treated during this ten-year period, for it depends on the criteria one uses for distinguishing the cases from other conditions. If one accepts "acroparesthesia"—as described by Putnam and Schultze in the last century—in which there was numbness, edema, and QEW test failure, then there were several hundred. But if one also requires, as a stipulation of the diagnosis, weakness in hand grip and some degree of weakness in the thenar muscles (at the base of the thumb), then the series of patients would be about twenty-five during this ten-year period.[10]

Thenar muscle atrophy, however, was *not* relieved by pyridoxine, although other signs and symptoms responded beautifully, and it took five months of treatment to relieve completely the cold perspiration in the palm of the secretary, L. S., who had been taking birth-control pills.

Because of the cases presented in this chapter, and other cases I have seen as well as investigations by others in the laboratory, the carpal tunnel syndrome can be definitely associated with a derangement in hormone metabolism. Two investigators, M. S. Sabour and H. E. Fadel, have reported a relation between the appearance of the carpal tunnel syndrome and the use of the antiovulatory contraceptive pills.[11] In their study, all sixty-two women studied improved within thirty days after contraceptive medication was discontinued; all of these patients had either the carpal tunnel syndrome (sixteen of whom had atrophy of the thenar muscles) or acroparesthesia. When fifteen of the patients subsequently resumed using the contraceptive pills, against medical advice, all fifteen experienced exacerbation of their symptoms again.

As we have seen in Case 1 in this chapter, L. S. had taken an antiovulatory contraceptive pill for ten years, and although the contraceptive pill was not discontinued, because of the patient's wishes, she responded to pyridoxine within three days. This indicates to me that the female hormone estrogen in the pill was probably the agent causing the carpal tunnel syndrome and that B$_6$ is important in the metabolism of estrogen.

S. M. Tobin in 1967 reported forty-two cases of carpal tunnel syndrome during pregnancy.[12] Again we have a time of life during which the female hormone estrogen is playing a far more dominant role than at other times. And, as we have seen in Case 2 in this chapter, the patient A. F. had extensive edema during pregnancy, and it responded to increased doses of pyridoxine. The same patient developed classical carpal tunnel syndrome three years after that, and this, too, responded to pyridoxine—within three days.

Dr. Max Wachstein, a distinguished pioneer in clinical studies of B$_6$ during pregnancy, has concluded that a relative vitamin B$_6$ deficiency exists during pregnancy.[13] David P. Rose has shown that contraceptive pills cause derangement of excretion of the urinary metabolites that are also associated with B$_6$ deficiency.[14] Thus we have a manifold increase in estrogen and other hormones during pregnancy, and the antiovulatory pills also account for an increase in estrogen. In turn, estrogen causes derangement in excretion of the same metabolites associated with B$_6$ deficiency. From this it follows that during these two times of life, certainly, the diet should be supplemented with B$_6$, for, as we have seen here, the carpal tunnel syndrome as associated with pregnancy and with contraceptive pills does respond to large doses of pyridoxine.

Although it will be examined more closely in subsequent chapters, it is worth noting that Phalen associated the carpal tunnel syndrome with diabetes and families that had a history of diabetes. Both of the patients, L. S. and A. F., in this chapter had relatives with diabetes. The Japanese scientist Yakito Kotake has indicated through animal research that xanthurenic acid, a metabolite of the amino-acid tryptophan, when increased in a B$_6$ deficient animal, can cause diabetes. Eclampsia, the convulsive disorder of pregnancy, is also far more common in the diabetic pregnant patient than in the rest of the pregnant population.

In cases involving pregnancy or the birth-control pills, in which the role of estrogen is obvious, it is easier to pinpoint what is probably happening in a patient's medical problems. In other cases the doctor is sometimes puzzled as to what exactly is going on.

One such case was that of M. W. During this ten-year period I never had another patient quite like him, and his condition was unique, at least in my experience, so that we, the authors of this book, were uncertain as to which chapter to put him in!

M. W., forty-two, was examined on February 8, 1970. His complaint: "I have a wart on my hand." Although he didn't have a lot of symptoms, he nonetheless had understated his problem considerably. A quite large man, six feet four inches tall and weighing 245 pounds, he had a verruca in the palm of his right hand, which was merely an incidental finding. I observed that his fingers in both hands were so disabled that he couldn't use his fingers as everyone else does. He couldn't hold packages, small boxes, or brooms with his right hand. In order to sweep, as he was required to do in the course of his job, he had to hold a broom handle with both palms pressed flat together around it. As I looked closely I saw that he had slight, but diffuse, edema in both hands and fingers. I showed him how to perform the QEW test. He couldn't flex his fingers properly for it.

As we discussed his case he explained that he had first had trouble with his hands and fingers at an early age. "I could never hold a pencil enough to write so I could read my own writing until I was nearly grown," he said. "I knew how to write, but I just couldn't hold the pencil right."

When he was sixteen he had tried to learn to milk a cow, which by then all of his brothers and sisters could already do, but he could never squeeze the teats sufficiently to produce milk in the pail. Yet, except for a siege of influenza about two months before I first saw him, he had had no serious illnesses or injuries. In fact, he was apparently normal except for his extremities, but there his failure to flex his fingers at the interphalangeal joints was so spectacular that I made motion pictures at the first examination for study later. The film recorded the wart in one palm, a reduced range and speed of flexion at the interphalangeal joints, and the peculiar way he held his pencil and wrote without using his fingers.

Strangely enough, despite his complex disability at the interphalangeal joints, he could still make a normal-appearing fist with both hands. There was little or no impairment in flexion of his fingers at the metacarpophalangeal joints. It was as if his trouble had either skipped those joints and gone on to the two outer finger joints, or as if the trouble had started at the outer joints of the fingers but had not yet reached the knuckles of the hand, or the metacarpophalangeal joints.

His case didn't fit in neatly with any other I have ever seen, but based on the fact that his hands were affected, I had him take 50 milligrams of pyridoxine daily from that day on.

The results were spectacular. On February 15, just seven days after beginning therapy, M. W. returned. Although he had been afflicted with most, if not all, of his disabilities since childhood, he showed heartening improvement in five areas. Considering the length of time he had suffered already, it would hardly be exaggerating to term his response *incredible*.

1. He now had complete flexion of all fingers at the interphalangeal joints, passing the QEW test.

2. He enjoyed more rapid flexion of his fingers.

3. There was more sustained power of flexion.

4. A visual inspection showed that the mild and diffuse edema of the hands had been eliminated.

5. Now, for the first time in memory, at age forty-two, he could write with a pen, using his index finger and his thumb in a normal manner! This is documented by a motion-picture film—irrefutable evidence, I would think.

On April 11, about two months following his first visit, I had occasion to observe M. W. in his home. Since beginning pyridoxine therapy he could use his hands much better in his work, he said, he could grip objects better, and he had no medical complaints. As I examined his hands he accomplished the QEW test with complete flexion, in a normal manner, of all fingers at the interphalangeal joints.

The mechanism of his recovery was as puzzling as the etiology of his disability, but whatever pyridoxine was doing, it was doing it right, and I advised him to take 50 milligrams daily as long as he lived.

As I have said, the authors placed M. W.'s case here, as the last one in this section on the carpal tunnel syndrome and rheumatism, because we were not sure exactly where the case did belong. M. W. did not have the classical symptomatology of rheumatism as I had come to recognize it. He never complained of paresthesia of the hands. He said he never had pain in shoulders, arms, or hands. Nocturnal muscle spasms never bothered him.

Of significance, however, was the fact that his wife had been troubled with paresthesia of the hands for six years. Her hands would "fall asleep" as if something like pins and needles were sticking into them. She had had muscle spasms in her legs at night. Her paresthesia and muscle spasms had been cleared up within six weeks by 50 milligrams of pyridoxine daily. It had taken her six times as long as it had him to improve markedly; yet she had had her signs and symptoms for a much shorter time than he had.

It is remarkable even to me—and I am usually not overly excited by B_6's speedy results—that M. W.'s flexion problems cleared up within seven days, although he apparently had had them practically a lifetime. For years he had either accepted his condition with resignation or, incredibly, did not know he should be getting more use from his hands. One can ponder these facts: As a child he couldn't hold a pencil in order to write. At sixteen he couldn't squeeze a cow's teats sufficiently to milk. Twenty-six years later he could barely flex his fingers, as if they were those of an old man in his last days. Yet within seven days, taking 50 milligrams of B_6 daily, he enjoyed normal, rapid, strong, and sustained finger flexion, readily breezing through the QEW test.

If one could visualize M. W. at age eighty and still untreated, I would expect to find him with sclerodactylia (a hardening of the fingers). His fingers would be stiff, insensitive and ineffective for purposes of perception, and virtually useless. I have seen borderline cases of sclerodactylia that were improved slightly by B_6 therapy, just enough to lead me to believe that sclerodactylia can be prevented with pyridoxine.

M. W.'s case is not only difficult to classify, but his swift recovery makes it exceptional. Although edema was frequently relieved in a matter of days, rarely did other signs and symptoms respond as soon as did M. W.'s problems. Other medical problems tended to have a slightly more protracted period of improvement. This apparently was because of more complicated patterns of signs and symptoms. For instance, those patients with long-standing acroparesthesia also had varying degrees of pain and loss of function of their shoulders and elbows. This "shoulder-hand syndrome" seemed definitely related to signs in the wrist and hand, but hand function could be restored more readily than could function of the elbows and shoulders. Long-standing edema and paresthesia of the hands would subside within three to six weeks when pyridoxine was used, but it might take several months before a patient suffering from painful shoulders could reach behind him or overhead. While there was dramatic improvement in shoulder signs and symptoms of some patients, as in that of the woman who tried to draw water from the well, relief of shoulder pain remained incomplete in others. On the whole, however, there was enough improvement in this syndrome to say that vitamin B₆ definitely improved it.

It seems likely to me that the shoulder-hand syndrome is also a part of the chronic derangement of steroid metabolism, is a late-stage development, and is, to a varying degree, irreversible in some persons. Yet it is responsive enough to B₆ for me to state emphatically that B₆ is necessary for both the prevention and the treatment of the shoulder-hand syndrome.

R. S. Phillips has reported that 17 percent of the cases he operated on for compression of the median nerve also had trigger finger.[15] In my own clinical experience, 300 to 400 milligrams of pyridoxine daily were sometimes necessary before there was noticeable improvement of trigger finger.

Heberden's nodes appear to be a part of periarthritis of the finger joints affecting women near the age of menopause. The redness of the newly formed Heberden's nodes tended to subside following treatment with pyridoxine (50 to 100 milligrams daily), and pain and swelling were reduced in the dense connective tissues adjacent to the Heberden's nodes. Once formed, however, the little bony excrescences tended to remain. In effect, then, pyridoxine was most effective in the early treatment of periarthritis of the interphalangeal joints and the accompanying Heberden's nodes, a condition known as menopausal arthritis. Eventually, it seems to me, the rheumatologists will accept vitamin B_6 in their armamentarium for relief and correction of acroparesthesia, the carpal tunnel syndrome, trigger finger, and rheumatism that were heretofore thought to be vague and ill-defined in the shoulder and elbow. There is no question but that a number of my patients also had periarticular swelling around the knees, with some fluid in the knees; as the rheumatism was relieved in the shoulders, arms, and hands, there also was a reduction of pain and swelling in the knees. The knees have not been commented on a great deal in this book for the simple fact that so many different things can happen to knees, ranging from injury to various diseases, consistently complicating the picture. More proof can be offered in the hands and shoulders.

Thus, while disturbances in the knees might be difficult to assess and even more difficult to trace or relate in etiology, those of the hands, especially, in the pertinent cases can be readily related to malfunctions in the nerves and muscles, as well as the skeletal system, as a result of hormonal and other imbalances. In these cases, the sometimes startling beneficial effect of vitamin B_6 is clearly evident.

Menstruation and Menopause | 5

One evening in July 1963, as I had just finished making my rounds at the hospital* and was returning the patients' charts to the rack, I noticed the puffed hands and fingers of the registered nurse on duty as she wrote at her desk. I had already had some clinical experience in relieving the edema of pregnancy with B$_6$ therapy, and therefore her hands, edematous, intrigued me.

"Do your hands ever tingle and go to sleep?" I asked.

D. O., the nurse, stopped writing and looked at me. "Yes, my hands go to sleep, and they not only go to sleep but they hurt. How did you know?"

"I didn't. I just wondered what you could tell me about them. You are a registered nurse; you might have observed some things about your hands that could help me understand why people's fingers swell and tingle."

She glanced over her shoulder and lowered her voice. "Dr. Ellis, there is something about this that has to do with my menstrual cycle. About midway between my periods is when I notice that the swelling and soreness begin. It lasts from seven to ten days and goes away when I menstruate."

* Titus County Memorial Hospital, Mt. Pleasant, Texas.

It seemed probable that what she had was premenstrual edema. For years gynecologists had been giving diuretics and hormones in attempts to control premenstrual edema and the so-called arthritis that was often associated with it. Because of other observations I had already made by then, I wondered if it might respond to B_6.

The next day D. O. came to my office to explore her problem further. At thirty-eight, she had regular menstrual periods, but during the past summer she had noticed swelling of her face, feet, and fingers. The swelling of her fingers was particularly noticeable because she had to remove her rings. All of her finger joints were sore, and the soreness was especially obvious while she was driving or typing. After a morning's activity, during which the hands were used normally, the swelling had subsided to the point where she could get her rings back on. She had learned that the swelling and soreness did not persist indefinitely. After a few days they would go away. As she became more aware of dates she began to associate them with her menstrual cycle.

She had taken a patented aspirin preparation, but nothing else, during the times she had the soreness, swelling, and pain. She thought the aspirin had reduced the aching in the joints some, but it had had no effect on the swelling. Furthermore, she didn't sleep well at night and would get up in the mornings stiff and sore all over. This was a pattern that she had noticed for several months. Once menstruation was completed, the swelling and soreness subsided, only to return later in the month. At the time of her office visit her fingers were swollen, and she said they were also sore and painful.

I prescribed two 50-milligram B_6 tablets daily for five days and asked her to return on the sixth day.

On the sixth day she reported: "After taking the B_6 for two days my hands were better—in fact, seemed well. By the third day I was able to wear my rings, use the typewriter, and sleep much better."

For the next twelve months she took one 50-milligram tablet daily and had no pain in her hands. Occasionally she would have a slight tightness in her hands but not enough to be apparent to the eye. During this time she had no premenstrual swelling, wore her wedding rings, and typed without soreness.

At this point, because of the expense and apparently because she thought daily pyridoxine was no longer necessary, she discontinued taking the tablets every day and began taking 50 milligrams on each of the ten days preceding menstruation. She had done this for four months when I next saw her, and it had been controlling her edema. Thus, in all, she had been taking B_6 for a period of sixteen months—a daily dose for one full year, a modified dose before menstruation for four months.

In order to make certain the pyridoxine was doing what we thought it was, I asked her to discontinue taking the tablets altogether. It was now October 1, 1964, and her next menstrual period was due on October 15.

Menstruation began, as expected, on October 15. She had no difficulty, noticed no symptom.

About a month later, however, on November 13, she developed a muscular soreness in the back of her neck that she described as a "crick." During that night she woke up with pain in her fingers and a general feeling of vague discomfort and a slightly depressed feeling. During the next day—November 14—she developed severe pains in the joints of her left hand, and she took two buffered aspirins. Her entire left hand was painful, while in the right hand only the distal interphalangeal joint of the index finger was involved. Her worst pain was in the ring and little fingers of the left hand. Unmistakably, she had edema in her face, hands, and fingers. Her fingers were so painful that she could hardly bear to lift the hospital chart with them.

Now she was frightened. "I can't be without the use of my fingers," she said. "I have to work. This is the worst spell I have ever had. I never had anything like this when I was taking the B_6."

On November 15, the next day, she began menstruating.

After this brief excursion back into a life without B_6 supplements, it was no problem to convince her of their effectiveness. During the next thirty days, of her own volition, she took 100 milligrams daily, beginning on November 16.

When I saw her next I made this notation in my records: "Patient seen December 15: she has no swelling whatsoever in her fingers and hands; she has no joint symptoms whatsoever in her fingers and hands; she has tiny wrinkles in skin of face, fingers, and hands; she is due to menstruate tomorrow."

The next notation: "Patient began menstruating December 16; otherwise symptom and sign free."

Three months later—on March 17, 1965, when menstruation was just starting—after she had taken 50 milligrams a day during that time, a physical examination disclosed that her wedding rings were loose on her fingers, her eyelids were wrinkled and normal (which is to say, not swollen), and the tendons showed on the backs of her hands, rippling beneath skin that was wrinkled, loose, and pliable—all objective evidence of complete freedom from premenstrual swelling.

D. O. had prevented, with pyridoxine, *premenstrual edema*. She took pyridoxine (50 milligrams daily) for the next seven years. In 1972 she had perfect flexion of all fingers—without recurrent edema.

Following this case I was soon able to prevent habitual and recurrent premenstrual edema in three other women, making a total of four cases in a relatively short span of time. For months before beginning B_6 therapy, the other three women had been taking diuretics, attempting to make their kidneys excrete the excess fluid that had caused the puffiness. Given pyridoxine, they found it to be effective, and it became their choice over the diuretics. One thirty-nine-year-old woman would gain five or six pounds during the few days before menstruation. When pyridoxine was taken daily throughout the monthly cycle, it would prevent the collection of this edema fluid.

Over the years as I saw more and more patients, edema of the hands during the premenstrual period could be linked with evidence of abdominal distension, involuntary muscle spasms of the legs and feet, and swelling of the eyelids and face. In one group of women I treated for those disorders, four out of eleven of them had previously taken diuretics for control of edema, with little success. But when they took 50 to 100 milligrams of pyridoxine daily, all their signs and symptoms were relieved after the first cycle menstruation. Yet I never mentioned the word *salt* to them nor made any effort to restrict fluids. Nor did I use diuretics at any time. Vitamin B_6 was the lone agent.

The hormonal influences in these cases are, of course, crucial, and because of them the natural processes of menstruation and menopause that occur to all women may bring their own unique physiological stresses. Some women fortunately experience these medical events without significant symptoms. Others suffer monthly from premenstrual edema, or swelling, and abdominal distension.

The older woman is frequently afflicted with a particular kind of rheumatism that has been labeled "menopausal arthritis." Probably a long-time vitamin deficiency leaves the body inadequately prepared for menopause, when there seems to be an increased need for B_6, and the same may be true for some patients during menstruation.

When William Heberden (1710–1801) described the painful little burrs, or knots, that appear on the sides of the finger joints, he brought to light one of the signs frequently encountered in menopausal arthritis. (Heberden's nodes are also found in men and may be related to signs and symptoms occurring before and after a heart attack. This will be discussed in Chapter 10.) These nodes, as reported in a preceding chapter, were responsive to pyridoxine if they were not long-standing. Age seemed to be the predominant factor. In an aged woman one could not expect the bony excrescences to disappear as they might in a woman around thirty-nine years of age. Dense tissues around the bony nodes seemed to be the site of improvement with reduction of pain.

Early in my work during the sixties I saw two classical patients who were nearing menopause and had been troubled for several months by these very bright-red, distinctly circumscribed nodes on the finger joints. In both cases the pain subsided and the redness disappeared within five weeks after therapy began. In the initial stages, then, Heberden's nodes related to hormonal change could be treated successfully. In later stages there was less certainty, although the patient usually did benefit in other ways.

The appearance of various related complaints is common near or past the age of menopause. Many of these disorders occur later in men, often during their sixties, there too suggesting a hormonal relationship. In the woman it may take the form of just slightly sore and stiff joints or it may be more serious. But in either type of case, as in all of the cases already presented and yet to be presented in this book, there is a common thread running throughout, and the thread can be identified by the various responses to pyridoxine in treatment.

In order to study in greater detail the complaints found around the age of menopause, let us look at the case of H. L. G., forty-seven, who had undergone a simple hysterectomy seventeen years before. Seen on September 19, 1962, she had "stiffness and soreness" in her finger joints, and a tingling numbness of her fingers and hands disturbed her sleep at night.

I could see that her fingers and hands had a puffy swelling with no wrinkles in the skin and no tendons visible on the dorsum of the hand. She could not flex the fingers of either hand to the metacarpophalangeal crease of the palm, as in the QEW test, and she winced at an ordinary handshake.

After two weeks of pyridoxine (50 milligrams orally a day), when I saw her on October 13 she was almost free of pain in her fingers and hands. She said the tingling and numbness had ceased in her fingers and hands during, and following, sleep. She completed the QEW test successfully, and the wrinkles of the skin, as well as the tendons, were conspicuous on the dorsum of the hands. She experienced no pain from an ordinary handshake, and she could rap her knuckles on a hard-topped desk without any unusual reaction. She was given pyridoxine for sixty days more; then it was discontinued. On March 25, 1965, when I saw her next, she showed a wrinkling on her hands and exhibited full flexion with no evidence of pain.

In the case of H. L. G., her discontinuing pyridoxine did not bring on a relapse, at least not in a relatively near time span. In other women, however, continued relief without B_6 did not last so long, indicating, as is found over and over in medicine, the significance of individual differences.

In many cases, the increased need for pyridoxine, once established, continued. One case, involving a woman who had "menopausal arthritis" (although she had not yet reached menopause), even contained features that might be termed a minor international incident. It demonstrates what frequently happens to a woman with "menopausal arthritis" when, following improvement, she discontinues taking pyridoxine.

The patient, J. C. P., thirty-nine, had painful, reddened Heberden's nodes near the distal finger joints of both hands when she was observed on February 15, 1965. She worked as a cosmetician, and the condition of her hands made her work very difficult. For the past six months she had suffered from numbness and tingling of the fingers and hands and could not touch or even approximate the right index finger to the thumb with enough strength to hold a pencil and write a letter. Bumping or squeezing of the finger joints gave her intense pain. Her left wrist and both shoulders were also painful. At night she had cramps in her leg muscles and would have to get out of bed to massage away the painful spasms. She had gained some relief by soaking her hands in hot water, but it aided her only temporarily. She complained of fluid collecting in her feet and legs, especially prior to menstruation; edema had been so marked during the preceding month, just before menstruation, that she had feared she would have to have her ring cut off the finger.

At the time of the first office visit, at which time I prescribed 50 milligrams of pyridoxine daily, she had the reddest Heberden's nodes that I have ever seen.

When she returned on March 9 she reported, "My fingers are not as stiff in the joints. I can move them better—can't you see?" She flexed all her fingertips to the metacarpophalangeal crease of the palm in a perfect demonstration of the QEW test and added, "My arms and hands don't go to sleep at night like they did, either."

The Heberden's nodes were still present on her finger joints, but they were less reddened and they weren't as painful to pressure.

On the first day of menstruation the following month, April 12, she had no edema in her hands, feet, or ankles, her ring was loose on her finger, and she rapped on a desk—painlessly—so hard with her knuckles that my secretary in the outer reception room heard her and thought someone was knocking on the door. The patient, J. C. P., had no swelling or pain in her hands and fingers except for a slight pain in the distal interphalangeal joints of the little fingers on full flexion. In her wrist and both shoulders the pain had subsided.

One year later, on March 28, 1966, when she was observed again, her hands were almost perfect. She had no pain. The Heberden's nodes had virtually disappeared. She performed the QEW test proficiently and readily. By then she had taken 50 milligrams of pyridoxine daily for a year.

Enter the international angle. That year her husband, a petroleum official, was sent by his company to Israel to work with the Institute for Petroleum Research and Geophysics in training Israelis to use seismographic equipment in oil exploration. On May 17, 1966, J. C. P. left by plane with her husband for Tel Aviv. In her baggage was a small bottle of pyridoxine tablets, one month's supply.

A few days later they arrived in Rehovet, Israel, a farming community about twelve miles from Tel Aviv.

In a month her pyridoxine tablets were used up and she did not bother to replace them, since she was doing well. Furthermore, if she had known it, she was probably getting a good "average" or "normal" amount of vitamin B_6 from her diet, for the couple ate lots of fresh fruits and vegetables. Eggplants and potatoes were the main vegetables, and oranges, apples, grapes, and dates the fruits. Although meat was more rare, they also had cheese, frozen fish, eggs, and some chicken. Presumably, if she had had a "normal" need for B_6 her diet would have supplied it. But we must remember that 2 or 3 milligrams a day is about all the B_6 one "normally" gets from food, and one cannot eat enough food to get more than 5 milligrams daily.

About six weeks after the B_6 tablets had been discontinued, complications began. She had a recurrence of the same complaints that she had suffered before, back in Texas more than a year previously.

"The little burrs on my fingers seemed to rise as if they had corruption in them," she said, "and I couldn't bring my index finger and thumb together enough to write with a pencil. My hands became numb and would tingle, and if I bumped them I was in great pain."

It was a crisis in her life and, therefore, in the life of her husband, for it interfered with his work.

"My husband told the Israeli officials to get me some vitamin B_6 tablets. No pyridoxine tablets could be found in Tel Aviv, and somebody went to Jerusalem and there were none there either. My daughter back in Texas sent me some vitamin B_6 tablets through the mail in some letters, but by the time the letters arrived the tablets were broken up into powder.

"It began to look hopeless.

"Finally, after about three months, my husband told the Israeli officials that if somebody didn't get some vitamin B_6 tablets over there for his wife he was going to take her back to the United States. The Israelis arranged things with customs, and the B_6 tablets were flown over and delivered to my front door."

That solved her crisis.

On January 4, 1972, J. C. P. was back in the United States, and I observed her again, by then nearly seven years since she had begun taking 50 milligrams a day. She did have Heberden's nodes, which were palpable and slightly tender, and she had a little pain in the joints of her fingers, but for all practical purposes she had full use and function of her hands. During her long bout with what apparently was either B_6 deficiency, or an increased need for B_6, J. C. P. had contributed a great deal of information. For one thing, as her case showed, the disorder among women that had been labeled "menopausal arthritis" wasn't very menopausal. Seven years after this crippling disease had first attacked her hands, she was still menstruating quite regularly. And she learned, over those seven years, that, at least as far as she was concerned, 100 milligrams of pyridoxine daily would control premenstrual edema better than 50 milligrams.

Much earlier, in the formative years of my work with B_6 in the clinic, it was my good fortune to meet Professor Jan Bonsma, head of the Department of Animal Science at the University of Praetoria in South Africa. He had the finest grasp of hormone balance in the cow of any person I ever heard of. After years of observation he had determined that excessive feeding of cattle, to produce fat, causes female hormonal changes to the point that young cows become less fertile or even sterile. As he studied a

heifer's, or young cow's, physical appearance b
unveil a pattern of hormonal reaction that was def
and permanent, and to a great extent dependen.
nutrition. He had demonstrated conclusively that cer..
of a cow were subject to female hormones found in cattle an.
these features were responsive to nutritional change. Knowing the
implications of comparative anatomy, I began to wonder if
hormones in a woman could be altered by nutrition.

Studies of my early patients, including those at the beginning
of this chapter, indicated that Bonsma's work also had implications in the human animal as well. Once I realized this, I delved
into technical works dealing with chemistry and physiology and
found that the hormone-mineral fluid balance relationship, which
concerned me in my pursuit of premenstrual edema, was almost
pieced together. It was an extremely complex matter having to do
with three ductless, or endocrine, glands: the pituitary, a small
pea-sized gland at the base of the brain; the sex glands (ovaries in
the female and testes in the male); and the adrenals, which are
about the size and shape of a small oyster and set just above the
kidneys.

The adrenals and the ovaries both produce some hormones that
are exactly the same. Since the male does not have ovaries, it
seems reasonable to expect him to depend almost entirely on his
adrenal glands for certain of these hormones so necessary for his
well-being. In the female, as the ovaries cease functioning she too
has to rely more on her adrenal glands for supporting hormones.
In the male, the testicle produces half as much estrogen as does
the female. Meanwhile, the pea-sized pituitary gland might be seen
as a supervisor of all the glands of both the male and the female.
In different ways these glands affect fluid balance in the body.

More and more as I studied it seemed that B_6 deficiency might
be disturbing utilization of the hormones and resulting in edema.
This remains to be proved, but if it is true, then B_6 deficiency is
capable of distorting fluid balance, mineral balance, and hormone
balance. One thing I was sure of was that Americans in great
numbers were, and are, walking around with from five to seven
pounds of excess fluid in their bodies. The fluid could be eliminated
with B_6. This suggested very strongly that great numbers of

Americans had experienced B$_6$ deficiency at some time in their lives.

In recent years many doctors have become alarmed about the excessive amounts of fluid that many persons have in their bodies for no apparent reason. In some instances the fluid has a relationship to a specific disease. If a person has chronic low-grade heart failure, he would have excessive fluid. Certain types of kidney disease cause patients to spill a lot of albumin in the urine, and that patient soon develops excessive fluid in his body. But in the vast majority of affected persons, there is no logical reason to explain those five to seven extra pounds of fluid. I now became convinced that this unexplained collection of mild clinical and subclinical edema fluid was caused by B$_6$ deficiency.

B$_6$ is very likely essential for support of the adrenal glands, but how, exactly, does it work? The hormones or steroids produced by the adrenals have been given a great deal of attention. The most famous work is that done with cortisone. Cortisone has been used extensively in the treatment of different kinds of arthritis. Actually, however, there have been thirty different steroids obtained from extracts of the adrenal gland. The well-known cortisone, then, was just one of thirty.

Another one of the thirty was aldosterone, which is of tremendous importance to water balance. If secreted in excessive amounts, aldosterone could cause too great a loss of calcium and potassium through the kidneys. This became a whirling puzzle. Because of the leg cramps and increase of edema in some of my patients I felt certain that B$_6$ was associated with a potassium relationship, but I didn't know whether my patients had edema because of a disturbed adrenal function or because of a disturbed exchange of sodium and potassium through the cell walls themselves.

One thing was indisputable: Edema had been relieved over and over without particular attention to either sodium or fluid intake. Somehow, B$_6$ had done it all. The question was, Does pyridoxine have a simple diuretic effect—or did these patients have advanced vitamin B$_6$ deficiency that was corrected by pyridoxine? (A diuretic is a chemical that acts on the tubules of the kidneys and causes the kidneys to pass more water as urine.) The question is yet to be finally resolved. What is certain is that if pyridoxine is not diuretic in the usual sense, then it must have a striking effect on intracellular biochemical exchanges, the exact nature of which is yet to be revealed. But the fact that associated neuropathies were simultaneously improved as edema subsided indicated that vitamin B_6 was having more than a simple diuretic effect.

The Birth-Control Pill | 6

By 1966 I had concluded that vitamin B_6 is intimately associated with metabolism of the female hormones, in that the hormones either require increased amounts of B_6 or become toxic in the absence of sufficient B_6. This became apparent not only in clinical work involving women during pregnancy and menopause but also with those using birth-control pills. Numerous women using oral antiovulatory pills for birth control have suffered edema and abdominal distension. Others have suffered more severe discomforts that were relieved by vitamin B_6.

As early as 1964 I had observed one patient who was experiencing a metabolic malfunction related to the birth-control pill. In November of that year D. N., the young woman, was found to have remarkable abdominal distension. Its onset had occurred shortly after she began the birth-control pills.* This was one of the first birth-control pills on the market. It was very strong. Its quantitative strength was later reduced by other pharmaceutical houses without a loss of contraceptive powers.

Two days in a row—November 17, 18—the patient received a vitamin B-complex injection that also contained 50 milligrams of

* Antiovulatory hormones: 5 milligrams norethynodrel and 0.075 milligrams mestranol.

pyridoxine. The swift reduction in abdominal distension was striking. On November 21 she was put on 50 milligrams of vitamin B_6 daily by mouth. I next saw her on February 11, 1965, the day after she had taken her last antiovulatory pill in preparation for menstruation on February 13. A physical examination revealed no swelling in the abdomen and no edema in the face, ankles, or feet. The following month, on March 8, she was again examined; while she had a very slight edema, it did not approach that which she had had before pyridoxine treatment. Again, on April 8, one day before menstruation, she had no abdominal distension.

Another patient of those days, B. H., thirty-four, already the mother of four children, was given the first type of birth-control pill marketed. This was on February 26, 1964, and it was probably the one with the greatest quantitative strength.*

She had difficulty with the pills from the beginning. "I only took six of those tablets," she said. "I nearly fainted when I took the first dose. The next day I felt a little better, but just felt awful. I had a bad taste in my mouth and I felt extremely tired and fatigued. I would feel worse in the mornings and then feel a little bit better in the afternoons. For the next six months I didn't take any more birth-control pills."

She had a history of severe leg cramps during pregnancy. Her toes "would draw down, especially the one next to the big toe." She added: "And when my last baby was born, while I was on the delivery table I had cramps in my legs so bad I could hardly stand it."

That August she was given a milder birth-control pill, containing a smaller dose of hormones.† Although the cramps returned to her legs at night, she continued taking the birth-control medication.

When I saw her on January 11, 1965, she complained of leg cramps "almost every night for the past five months." At this time she was told to take 50 milligrams of pyridoxine daily, and by January 21, ten days later, she had had only one episode of leg cramps during that period. By March 16, about two months later, she reported: "My legs don't cramp and my ankles don't swell like they did before my periods."

---

* 9.8 milligrams norethynodrel and 0.15 milligrams mestranol.
† Norethindrone 1 milligram and mestranol 0.08 milligrams.

In a follow-up I discussed her physical condition with her on March 4, 1972, by which time she had been on birth-control pills —and vitamin B_6—for seven years, and she was taking both with comfort and satisfaction.

It was on the basis of these cases, and other observations, that I wrote in 1966, concerning this altered balance of steroids: "There is powerful evidence to indicate that B_6 starvation, pre-existing, is directly associated with conspicuous edema of pregnancy, of the premenstrual period, and the use of antiovulatory drugs."[1] Later that year, after my autobiographical book had been published in June, I met Dr. Paul György, the discoverer of vitamin B_6, and Dr. David B. Coursin, one of the clinical pioneers in the history of B_6, both of whom appeared in Chapter 2. On December 28, 1966, in company with Dr. György and Dr. Coursin at the Faculty Club of the University of Pennsylvania School of Medicine, I reported my observations concerning B_6 and the antiovulatory pill to both the corporate director and the medical director of Hoffmann-La Roche, the drug company. My patients had already provided enough clinical support to point toward the need for increased B_6 in women taking oral contraceptives. Since that time Hoffmann-La Roche and others have done the laboratory work to bear out the earlier clinical recognition of the disorder. In 1966 David P. Rose presented his paper which in the laboratory supported the same conclusion. Dr. Rose did his work at Sheffield University in England.[2]

Realizing that there was a relationship of the female hormones and B_6, I still was not sure in my own mind just which one was implicated until 1969 when I attended the New York Academy of Sciences symposium on "Vitamin B_6 in Metabolism of the Nervous System." It was there that Merle Mason, Ph.D., a University of Michigan biochemist, and R. R. Brown, Ph.D., a University of Wisconsin chemist, told me that laboratory evidence had singled out estrogen as the female hormone requiring increased amounts of B_6.

Since 1966, research done by others has validated these earlier conclusions. Dr. A. Leonard Luhby and other researchers at the New York Medical College have shown that women on birth-control pills need up to 30 milligrams of vitamin B_6 daily in order

to bring to normal the excretion of xanthurenic acid in tι.
Dr. Myron Brin of Hoffmann-La Roche laboratories has statε
greater B_6 needs have been found "in up to 75 percent oι
women on oral contraceptives tested by us." He added that therε
was some suggestion that a B_6 deficiency either in pregnancy or
with the use of the Pill could lead to mental depression, although
the final evidence wasn't yet in. Birth-control pills, the Luhby-Brin
team reported, cause a metabolic condition in a woman's body that
resembles pregnancy, a time of life when B_6 requirements are accelerated.

Other researchers, including J. M. Price and his associates, have
shown that women taking oral contraceptives excrete an excessive
amount of xanthurenic acid when given the tryptophan-load test.
The biochemical change was reversed by the administration of
pyridoxine. In the British medical journal *Lancet*, M. J. Baumblatt
and P. Winston reported in 1970 that some of the symptoms associated with depression induced by oral contraceptives were
abolished by pyridoxine.[3] The *American Journal of Obstetrics and
Gynecology* has furthermore reported that birth-control pills con-
tribute to the carpal tunnel syndrome. The syndrome was relieved
by discontinuing birth-control pills. Chapter 4, "Rheumatism and
the Carpal Tunnel Syndrome," has already examined a case in
which the woman patient on antiovulatory pills developed the
carpal tunnel syndrome, which was relieved by vitamin B_6. A detailed exploration of these investigations of this medical problem
will be found in Chapter 11.

In summary, it is my recommendation that every woman who is
on birth-control pills should also take 50 to 100 milligrams of
pyridoxine daily.

B₆ During Pregnancy | 7

All pregnant women have an increased need for vitamin B₆.

During my clinical experience with vitamin B₆ I have attended 225 pregnant women who received B₆ therapy. Numerous signs and symptoms appear during pregnancy that are responsive to B₆. These include painful neuropathies in the fingers and hands, swelling (edema) in the hands and feet, leg cramps, hand and arms "that go to sleep," and, most of all, B₆ is a factor in the prevention and treatment of toxemia of pregnancy and the convulsions of eclampsia.

Edema—present in at least *one-third* of all pregnant women in the United States and England—is one of the most worrisome of signs to the obstetrician, because he fears it may, though not necessarily, presage toxemia of pregnancy, a form of poisoning that may threaten life of the mother or fetus or both. Toxemia, in turn, may be a step toward eclampsia, or convulsions, which is probably the most feared condition of pregnancy. In all likelihood there is no situation that may arise in pregnancy and delivery that frightens the obstetrician more than convulsions in pregnant women. It is a life-and-death situation, and one cannot be certain of the outcome.

In most pregnancies the growth of the fetus progresses to term, and normal birth follows, with the baby healthy and crying spontaneously. In such cases the mother has no complications. The majority of the 225 women I have attended in pregnancy fit this category. However, in order to pinpoint the medicinal effects of vitamin B6, I will be concentrating on cases that were not quite normal or that deviated widely from the normal. In order not to distort the general pattern that actually existed, it is necessary to emphasize that the cases used in this chapter are for the purposes of illustration and do not reflect the general trend.

It is accepted by now that proper nutrition is more important during pregnancy than at any other time. For this reason, any woman who suspects that she may be pregnant should check in with her physician immediately so that he can advise her on her nutritional obligations to herself and to her unborn child. He will insure that she is instructed as to a balanced diet that contains sufficient minerals and vitamins as she "eats for two," and he will prescribe vitamin-mineral supplements. As we will be seeing, sufficient vitamin B6 supplements will play an essential role during the nine months following conception.

Laboratory evidence as to the increased need for B6 during pregnancy is well established. Dr. Paul György has pointed out that all pregnant women studied have presented laboratory data that indicated additional B6 was necessary to normalize the excretion of certain metabolites in the urine. Specifically, based on the work of Dr. Max Wachstein, an early researcher, this refers to the excretion of xanthurenic acid, a metabolite of tryptophan, one of the essential amino acids. Tryptophan, the principal amino acid in meat, is involved in four different chemical reactions before it is excreted through the kidneys as xanthurenic acid. On the other hand, if the same amino acid, tryptophan, were to go through a different series of changes, it would form nicotinic acid, a factor useful in the treatment of pellagra. Thus, in one chain reaction, B6 and nicotinic acid are complementary. Much of the laboratory B6 data is based on the excretion of xanthurenic acid and other amino-acid metabolites in the urine. Both Wachstein, writing in the *American Journal of Clinical Nutrition* in 1956, and E. W. Page, in the *Western Journal of Surgery* in 1956, pointed toward an increased need for B6 during pregnancy.

Any woman who has ever been pregnant will confirm the statement that pregnancy brings more changes to the body than at any other time of life. Hormones that are hardly noticed at other times become active. New life, which was once a microscopic, germlike egg, is growing within the body of a human being. Each day, each month of its life, the fetus makes additional demands on its mother's body. From the moment of conception until the umbilical cord is severed at birth nine months later, the mother's body is constantly changing, constantly accommodating itself to the stress of producing another human being.

In these 225 cases from which I will be taking several for illustrative purposes, approximately 20 percent of the patients were Afro-American, 3 percent Latin American, and the remaining 77 percent Anglo-American. The majority came from the middle- or low-income groups. Some were unwed; the husband of one was in jail at the time. The series of 225 deliveries included six sets of twins, as well as breech births and those in which the baby's weight was less than five pounds, classifying it as "premature," and other unrelated complications of pregnancy. The infant mortality was below 2 percent. Maternal mortality was 0.

It is necessary to say that there was no apparent evidence of toxicity from pyridoxine among the 225 patients, although up to 1,000 milligrams a day were given in divided doses for short intervals of two to three days in some patients, without apparent ill effect on either mother or infant.

A theory has been given wide currency in obstetrical circles that water retention caused by excessive salt in the diet leads to swelling during pregnancy. To counteract this edema, it has become common practice for many obstetricians to restrict salt intake and to prescribe diuretics to pregnant women who show signs of such swelling. In these 225 cases, *no effort was made to restrict salt in any of the patients, and none of the women received a diuretic.* In fact, the word *salt* was never mentioned, and the patient's diet was rarely altered or even discussed. There is no reason for salt restriction during pregnancy; in fact, there more likely is a danger in restricting it. A certain amount of salt is necessary for proper electrolyte exchange, and, after all, it is not the primary cause of edema in the first place, as we will see. Furthermore, if salt had been restricted, critics would have claimed that salt restriction was important in the prevention of convulsions; this, as we will see, is not true.

The need for salt during pregnancy has been recognized by the White House Conference on Food, Nutrition, and Health, which I attended in 1969. At that time a formal statement was made by the conference to this effect: "Sodium retention is, in fact, a normal physiological adjustment during pregnancy, and is directly related to normal blood volume expansion and tissue growth. If dietary sodium is limited, there is increased stimulation of the normal sodium conservation mechanisms. The resulting increase in aldosterone secretion increases the quantity of sodium reabsorbed from the kidney filtrate. Sodium restriction observed in laboratory animals produces extreme enlargement and even exhaustion of the aldosterone-secreting cells of the adrenal cortex. Examination of the fine structure of these cells indicates extreme pathology when animals are subjected to the double stress of sodium restriction and pregnancy."

The statement went on to term "promiscuous use of diuretics" during pregnancy as "antagonistic" to the physiological adjustment and worsening the stress on the salt-conserving mechanism. It concluded by recommending a re-examination of sodium requirements during pregnancy, noting that laboratory evidence suggested an increased need for salt. Finally it said that diuretics during the normal pregnancy "should not be condoned."

Some of my patients were given a vitamin-mineral supplement plus increased amounts of B₆, while others were given pyridoxine alone. It is granted that B₆ alone is not the only answer to proper nutrition during pregnancy, and I do not intend to indicate this in any way.

When I first began to use B₆ in treating pregnant patients I feared that the safety of both mother and fetus might require a low dosage. For this reason I used prenatal capsules, produced by different pharmaceutical companies, that were well accepted in the medical profession. These were multivitamin-mineral supplements containing from 3 to 10 milligrams of pyridoxine, depending on the particular brand. One capsule was given daily.

The 10 milligrams seemed to be sufficient for many of the patients, but it soon became evident that 3 to 10 milligrams of pyridoxine daily were not enough to relieve a number of symptoms, especially swelling in the hands and feet of a number of pregnant women. At that point, larger doses were given, and particular attention was given to changes in signs and symptoms within seventy-two hours after increasing the dose.

Of the signs and symptoms often associated with pregnancy, several involve the nerves. Many disturbances of cell chemistry are first noticed in the nerves, and this pays tribute to the fact that the chemistry involved in the metabolic use of a vitamin must be truly fantastic. The nervous system is the first to respond to most chemical or organic changes, and for this reason one should logically expect vitamin B_6 or other deficiency to alter the nervous system's function. Because of this, nerve function has been very useful in studying vitamin B_6 in the clinic. Leg cramps, paresthesia of the hands, and painful finger joints in pregnant women—all signs involving the nerves—responded to pyridoxine, as had been the case with men and with non-pregnant women.

Occasionally a patient reported that an entire arm seemed to be paralyzed on awakening in the morning. The other hand would have to be used to shake or massage that arm in order to get it to function. *This transitory paralysis of an entire arm came to be considered a pathognomonic sign of increased need for vitamin B_6.* (Pathognomonic is a medical term for that which is characteristic of a disease, distinguishing it from other diseases.) Just as in the non-pregnant patients, pyridoxine would relieve the condition. Other patients suffered from pain in the interphalangeal joints of the fingers until administered from 50 to 450 milligrams of pyridoxine daily.

Leg cramps are a frequent complaint among pregnant women—often interpreted as a calcium deficiency. However, I was to observe some of the worst leg cramps in women who had been taking high quantities of calcium. Their leg cramps were not relieved until they also began taking B_6. When in rare instances pyridoxine alone failed to relieve foot and leg muscle spasms during pregnancy, the addition of potassium as an oral daily supplement usually eliminated muscle spasms completely. In recent years I have had a high degree of success in adding magnesium supplements to the therapy during the prenatal period.

A good example is that of E. M. H., thirty-nine, in her eighth pregnancy. Her mother was a diabetic, and on one occasion E. M. H.'s urine specimen contained sugar.

"My fingers and legs hurt and sometimes I have to work an hour to get the feeling back into my fingers," she said when she reported in for the first time. She was given a prenatal vitamin-mineral capsule that included 10 milligrams of pyridoxine. One month later she returned with her feet and legs more swollen, and now she complained of severe muscle spasms in her legs at night. Obviously, that amount of pyridoxine was insufficient. This time I prescribed 50 milligrams of pyridoxine daily in addition to that in the capsule.

By the third night, muscle spasms in the legs had subsided; within fourteen days she had lost eleven pounds, and the skin on the dorsum of her feet was wrinkled. The painful interphalangeal joints of her fingers were much improved, and the numbness, tingling, and impaired sensation in her fingers were eliminated. The clincher came when she reported, "My wedding ring got so loose I would lose it in the dishwasher. It is looser than it has been in years." This is objective evidence of relief from swelling, which we will be seeing over and over.

Although her blood pressure was 170/100—high—when she entered the hospital, her urine was negative for sugar and albumin, and her eight-and-one-half-pound son was born by breech birth and cried spontaneously.

For many years obstetricians have recognized that soon after the beginning of pregnancy women are likely to drop objects, usually dishes. What is involved here is a failure of neuro-muscular coordination of hand and finger flexion, and the reason for it had been unknown. *Pyridoxine relieved dropping of objects during pregnancy in these patients.*

Such symptoms were experienced by the second pregnant patient I treated with pyridoxine, back in 1962. She was a twenty-one-year-old Negro woman who was eight months pregnant.

"When I pick up things with my right hand," she explained, "I drop them, and every time I write, my hand goes to sleep. My husband is in the service, and when I try to write him, my hand goes to sleep and then it starts paining me."

At that time, early in my work with B_6, I was giving pyridoxine hydrochloride by injection. Every other day for two weeks she came to the office for 50 milligrams given by needle into the deltoid muscle of the upper arm.

At the end of the injections the patient was much improved. "Two weeks ago I was apt to drop a plate if I picked it up," she said. "Now I can hold the plate. Before the shots my arm would feel asleep and numb and would have a 'sticking' like pins and needles in it. I haven't had the pins and needles sticking in my arm since the second shot [given on the third day]. I still had a little numbness in my right fingers today when I picked up a dough-nut. Before taking the shots I could hold my umbrella but then couldn't straighten out my fingers without rubbing them. Now I can hold it and then straighten out my fingers, but they feel a little numb. Before, I had to hang my arm over the side of the bed so I could sleep because of hurting and feeling numb; now I can lie with it in the bed beside me. I still have that dizzy-headedness."

To this patient, as with all of the others discussed in this chapter, I never mentioned salt. Yet she experienced a spectacular reduction of edema in her hands and feet, along with the improved coordination of her hands. As the puffy swelling disappeared, tiny, faint wrinkles developed in the skin of her hands and feet. At the end of two weeks the wrinkles were remarkably conspicuous.

At first glance this momentary transitory paralysis of a hand, as we term the condition of women dropping dishes during pregnancy, may not seem important. But consider the possible effect on the nervous system that is being developed in the unborn child.

As we come to a full-scale discussion of edema in pregnancy, we come to a common discomfort and hazard. As mentioned, one-third of the pregnant American women, and one-third of the pregnant English women, suffer swollen hands and feet during pregnancy. They may also have neuritis and neuropathies, and some even have the carpal tunnel syndrome, a disabler at the wrist discussed in Chapter 4. The Negro woman who was having trouble writing with a pencil was developing the carpal tunnel syndrome until given pyridoxine.

Edema of pregnancy, long discussed in both medical and lay circles, has become so common that many doctors have come to accept it as being normal during pregnancy, and patients have grown resigned to suffering through it. *It is not normal at all. It is not normal at any time.* The patient feels bad. There is nothing healthy about being swollen with fluids.

Based on my investigations with 225 pregnant women on B₆ therapy, in most cases vitamin B₆ will completely relieve and prevent edema of pregnancy as it has been known to the scientific community. This is a large statement, but it has been proved over and over. Because of the skepticism that some readers may entertain, it would be wise to repeat that in these 225 cases *no diuretics were given to any patient, and there was no restriction on either salt or fluids.*

Interestingly, in 1962, 50 milligrams of B₆ were far beyond the usually accepted nutritional demands during pregnancy. Several of my patients had been taking prenatal vitamin-mineral preparations before they developed edema. One capsule contained no pyridoxine, one had 5 milligrams, and another contained 10 milligrams. Yet, as pregnancy approached term, even 50 milligrams was inadequate to control edema in nine out of sixteen cases in one study series I conducted. Five of these nine were then controlled by increasing the pyridoxine oral dosage to 100 milligrams daily. The remaining four of the nine required injections of 150 milligrams daily, three of whom also received injections of B-complex vitamins. Two of the four requiring 150 milligrams by injections delivered normal twins—on the surface a logical explanation of their heightened need for the vitamin. In all of these cases, edema of the hands was controlled.

Other facts in these sixteen cases are of interest. Nine were primiparas, or women pregnant for the first time. Three, who were under twenty years of age, developed hypertension, with their highest recorded blood pressures at 180/120, 170/110, and 170/118. No antihypertensive drugs were given, and yet none had convulsions. (The only time I gave an antihypertensive drug was a case in another series, to be discussed in this chapter.)

Maternal weight control during pregnancy was related proportionally to control of edema. Weight changes in some instances were striking. One nineteen-year-old expectant mother in her first pregnancy lost thirteen pounds in seven days after receiving 150 milligrams of pyridoxine daily. One lost eight pounds in twelve days. Another responded but little to 50 milligrams; when pyridoxine was increased to 150 milligrams she lost fifteen pounds in eighteen days. One patient enjoyed a reduction in weight, then gained no weight during the last five weeks of pregnancy, for a total of twenty pounds gained during the entire gestation period. These patients had marked edema of the hands and feet prior to receiving 150 milligrams daily. At the time of parturition they all demonstrated remarkable wrinkling of the skin on the dorsum of the hands and feet—normal signs.

Of these 225 cases, six patients required B complex plus pyridoxine by injection. Either these six patients were not absorbing oral pyridoxine properly or else they needed other B vitamins for the full benefit. Included in this group, as an example, was a child bride, fifteen years old when she married. Although 100 milligrams of pyridoxine daily by mouth relieved her edema for a while, the swelling returned. Thereafter three injections on alternate days of B complex with 100 milligrams of pyridoxine relieved the edema completely in the hands, and although there remained slight edema in the feet, there was a wrinkling in the skin of the feet.

In medicine, as perhaps in all other things, individuality is always important. Although a pattern may suggest lines of treatment that will benefit, let us say, nine out of ten patients, we always recognize that each patient's reaction may be different from the next. We never know which will be the tenth one that will be different.

From this observation we might assume that a woman maintaining a level of B$_6$ would be more likely to enter pregnancy without complications than one who was deficient from the beginning. This appears to be true generally. The difficult part is in ascertaining what are the daily needs of a particular individual. One person's daily B$_6$ requirement may be vastly different from another's for a number of reasons. But the case of V. H., at twenty-six in her third pregnancy, does show in one person what can be done in correcting the nutritional imbalance during a pregnancy and how preventive medicine, in the form of vitamin therapy, can insure relatively smooth sailing, medically speaking.

V. H. was seen for prenatal care on June 15, 1968, approxi-

mately three months pregnant. Prescribed a vitamin-mineral capsule and pyridoxine tablets that gave her a total of 175 milligrams
of B$_6$ daily, she complained of headaches in the fourth month of
pregnancy. The headaches had persisted for two weeks when she
reported them. Pyridoxine was increased to a total of 225 milligrams. The headaches subsided.

Beginning with the fifth month of pregnancy, she had swelling,
numbness, and tingling in the hands and feet. Pyridoxine was increased to 325 milligrams to relieve these symptoms. During the
sixth month her elbows and knees became painful, and sensation
was lost in the fingertips. She couldn't feel the heat of a match, and
on two occasions her fingers had been burned. Nor could she distinguish the texture of objects such as glass or wood. Because
of a failure in her hand grip she had difficulty grasping and holding
the handles of pots, pans, and other cooking utensils. On September 24 her feet had become more swollen, with a pitting edema
that clinically was recorded as 3-plus.

Because of these changes I raised her pyridoxine dosage to 425
milligrams daily. Seven days later, on October 1, all edema had
subsided, her hand grip was back to normal, the pain at flexion
of her fingers had ceased, and her fingertip sensation had returned
to normal. The increased dosage of pyridoxine continued until
December 13, at which time she entered the hospital wearing her
wedding rings and with no evidence of edema and no albumin or
sugar in her urine. The only departure from normal was that her
blood pressure was high, reading 160/90.

She delivered a six-pound, nine-ounce infant female who cried
spontaneously.

When she was discharged from the hospital I instructed her to
continue taking 50 milligrams of pyridoxine night and morning, a
total 100 milligrams daily, for an indefinite period.

The sequel to this pregnancy is interesting in what it tells us of
preventive medicine.

While still taking 100 milligrams of pyridoxine daily the patient
V. H. became pregnant again, and at the third month of pregnancy the same vitamin-mineral capsule was given as before, plus
an additional 100 milligrams of pyridoxine night and morning.
This provided her with a daily total of 225 milligrams.

There was no comparison of the two pregnancies. In the second one, after having been on B₆ before getting pregnant and on 225 milligrams since the third month, she continued to term—free of the symptoms she had suffered in the earlier pregnancy. No edema, no loss of hand grip, no numbness, tingling, or pain in the interphalangeal joints of the fingers. On January 19, 1970, a normal male infant was delivered. One month later, on February 19, I examined the mother and her two smallest children, and they were all apparently normal.

This was a relatively mild case of complications compared to some that obstetricians encounter in this country. V. H., in her earlier pregnancy, did not reach the stage of toxemia, one of the most dreaded conditions of pregnancy. Toxemia is usually preceded by edema, and this is why most obstetricians grow concerned when a pregnant woman becomes greatly swollen. Of toxemia, "a disease of civilization," Dr. Jack A. Klieger and associates have written: "We are blundering along today much as we did fifty years ago, with no precise idea as to its etiology and with treatment which, while rational, is anything but definitive." He classified the obtaining of information on the genesis of toxemia as "one of the greatest challenges in the entire field of human reproduction."[1] Since edema may be a prelude to toxemia, physicians in the past were fast to prescribe diuretics in an effort to reduce edema. Edema has been the leading, constant, and continually puzzling condition of pregnancy. In the next several cases we will be discussing, the patients went into the delivery room without having had either antihypertensive drugs or diuretics at any time they were under my care. Therapy was limited to vitamin B₆, in some cases combined with therapeutic doses of the minerals magnesium and potassium.

Probably most physicians follow a rule similar to mine—that when the diastolic blood pressure is 90 and when the systolic reaches 150 or more, I start worrying. Years ago the late Dr. Willard Cook, professor of obstetrics and gynecology at the University of Texas School of Medicine, cautioned nurses to watch carefully the obstetrical patient with an approaching systolic blood pressure of 160 because that patient would be likely to convulse. Hypertension is one of the standards by which toxemia of pregnancy is established clinically. When a patient has high blood pressure, is edematous, and has albumin in the urine, she can be said to have toxemia. If in addition to these signs she convulses, then she has eclampsia.

L. A., twenty-one and in her first pregnancy, weighed 140 pounds at the time of her first prenatal examination on June 15, 1968. She was more than three months pregnant then, and she was given a prenatal vitamin-mineral capsule with 10 milligrams of pyridoxine in it. To this I added 100 milligrams, to provide 110 milligrams a day. On August 25, slightly over two months later, I substituted another capsule that would provide 25 milligrams of B6, which in all gave her 125 milligrams daily. The capsule also contained 100 milligrams of magnesium oxide and 1 milligram of magnesium sulfate.

On October 11 she noticed extensive swelling of her hands and feet, and I increased her pyridoxine intake to 425 milligrams daily. One week later she had marked pitting edema of the feet and legs and, for the first time, 4-plus albuminuria and a blood pressure of 170/90. She had gained eight pounds in seven days, sending her weight up to 183 pounds. Her hands were so swollen that her fingers could hardly be flexed enough to make a fist. She complained of numbness, tingling, and pain in her fingers. Sensation in her fingers was impaired. She had distinct pain in her proximal and distal interphalangeal joints.

On three successive days—October 22, 23, and 24—she received injections of an additional 500 milligrams of pyridoxine into the deltoid muscle of the shoulder. This meant that during this three-day period she received 925 milligrams daily, or a total of 2,775 milligrams.

By October 25, seventy-two hours after the injections had begun, the edema had subsided in the hands, wrinkles could be seen on the dorsum of the hands, and there was considerable reduction of edema in the feet.

The following day, October 26, she was admitted to the hospital in active labor, with no detectable edema in the hands and only slight edema in her feet. Her blood pressure was 170/90, and she had a 4-plus albuminuria. After five hours of labor a six-pound, one-and-one-half-ounce infant male was born, crying spontaneously and appearing normal. L. A., the mother, had been given 100 milligrams of pyridoxine by intramuscular injection on admission to the hospital and 100 milligrams every twelve hours thereafter until discharged on October 28. Her blood pressure at 7:00 A.M. the day after delivery was 166/100. On the morning of her discharge from the hospital, slightly over a day after giving birth, her urine was negative for albumin, and a microscopic examination revealed no casts. By November 14, slightly over two weeks later, her blood pressure was down again, to 120/80.

Patient L. A. had met the criteria necessary for a diagnosis of toxemia of pregnancy. She had an elevated blood pressure, severe albuminuria distinct from that of nephritis or inflammation of the kidney, and she had edema in the prenatal period. Pyridoxine had controlled her edema, and although it had had no influence on her prenatal hypertension she had proceeded uneventfully to term delivery.

The addition of potassium and magnesium has been a part of the therapy of a number of patients. In the latter part of my clinical studies, magnesium became a frequent part of the treatment.

C. S., in her first pregnancy at nineteen, was first admitted to the hospital on January 18, 1970, suffering from severe nausea, vomiting, and dehydration associated with the first trimester of pregnancy. She was hospitalized for four days, and her treatment consisted primarily of intravenous fluids containing electrolytes and multivitamins that included pyridoxine. Vomiting subsided, and as she left the hospital she was instructed to take 50 milligrams of pyridoxine morning and night, along with a prenatal capsule of vitamins and minerals that included 25 milligrams of pyridoxine, 100 milligrams of magnesium oxide, and 1 milligram of magnesium sulfate. This patient was especially watched closely because she had a sister who was a diabetic taking insulin. Because of a tendency of diabetes to run in families, the physician is understandably cautious in treating a patient with a diabetic close relative.

For the following several months, then, she took 125 milligrams of pyridoxine daily. On July 15, nearly six months after hospitalization, extensive edema developed in her hands and feet. Pyridoxine was increased to 325 milligrams daily, and within seventy-two hours all edema had completely subsided in the hands and feet. Her urine continued to be negative for albumin and sugar, and her blood pressure was 120/78.

On September 23 she had a recurrence of edema in her hands and feet. This time the pyridoxine dosage was not increased but kept at 325 milligrams daily, while 1,000 milligrams each of potassium aspartate and magnesium aspartate were added. Three days later, on September 26, she was admitted to the hospital in active labor and with evident medical problems. Her blood pressure was 166/100, her catheterized urine specimen showed 4-plus albuminuria, and she was quite apprehensive. She had slight tremors of the hands.

At 6:00 A.M. she was given 40 milliequivalents of potassium gluconate by mouth, which was almost immediately vomited. She was also given 200 milligrams of pyridoxine by intramuscular injection. By 6:45 A.M. she had remarkably, definitely relaxed. Without sedatives the tremors of her hands had subsided, and she slept soundly between labor contractions, even though the cervix was dilated 8 centimeters—to a significant degree.

Her restful intermittent relaxation continued until 8:00 A.M., when for the first time she complained of a headache. Blood pressure was then 160/120. By 8:10 A.M. the cervix was completely dilated, and at 9:44 A.M. a normal infant was delivered, crying spontaneously.

The nurse's and physician's notes agreed that forty-five minutes after the 200-milligram injection of pyridoxine the patient C. S. was much calmer, much more relaxed, and dozing between contractions. Subsequent 200-milligram injections were given at 9:15 A.M., 12:30 P.M., and midnight. Two weeks after delivery the mother exhibited no albuminuria, and her blood pressure was back to normal.

Again, the criteria had been met for a diagnosis of toxemia. C. S. had had a marked elevation of blood pressure, a 4-plus albuminuria, and edema. Edema had been partially controlled by pyridoxine in the prenatal period and finally controlled by 800 milligrams given during the twenty hours during which parturition occurred. It is no doubt significant that she was given 3,000 milligrams of magnesium aspartate and 3,000 milligrams of potassium aspartate during the seventy-two-hour period before she went into labor. It might be emphasized that C. S. very likely had a reasonably normal electrolyte balance of magnesium and potassium on admission to the hospital. Thus the stage was set for the optimum effect of the two co-factors, pyridoxine and magnesium.

Our discussion of edema and toxemia logically leads into the most dangerous condition of pregnancy, and that is what is meant by the medical term *eclampsia*. Edema often presages toxemia. Toxemia may lead into eclampsia.

What is eclampsia? While still a medical student I saw a memorable case of eclampsia in a Houston hospital. This Negro woman had hands swollen puffy like a balloon. The doctors attending her were so afraid she would go into convulsions and die that they had her asleep with barbiturates, which was the best way they knew to prevent her from convulsing.

When an eclamptic patient starts convulsing she loses consciousness, and there is a generalized shaking like that of a dog poisoned with strychnine. The woman may bite her tongue, or she may, in a sense, swallow her tongue and choke to death. The convulsions may go away and then come back with another general *grand mal* seizure.* Some women have been known to have only one—and die. In less severe cases the convulsive seizures are lighter and are characterized by tonic and clonic tremors of arms and legs.

In a diagnosis of true eclampsia, three things are necessary. The patient must have albuminuria (albumin in the urine), hypertension, and convulsions. As soon as albuminuria and hypertension appear, the physician is warned to start trying to head off convulsions, the deadly third condition of eclampsia.

Laboratory data by Wachstein indicated that B$_6$ would favorably influence eclampsia. In pioneer work at St. Catherine's Hospital in New York he had concluded in 1956 that 10 milligrams of vitamin B$_6$, given daily, would favorably influence the incidence of pre-eclampsia that might lead to convulsions. However, Dr. Wachstein was a pathologist and did not have the opportunity to study the effects of B$_6$ in the obstetrical suite. He was basing his decisions on

---

* A sudden unconsciousness associated with violent contraction of all voluntary muscles to produce rigid stiffness of arms, legs, back, and neck.

metabolites excreted in the urine before and after treatment with pyridoxine. He paved the way for much of my work.

In my opinion, 300 to 400 milligrams of pyridoxine a day, administered with 1,000 milligrams of magnesuim oxide or aspartate and 1,000 milligrams of potassium aspartate, will prevent both edema and eclampsia—unless the patient has diabetes. The B_6 plus magnesium and potassium represent, primarily, prophylaxis against convulsions. Unless one is dealing with a frank diabetic, such therapeutic use of B_6, magnesium, and potassium will, I am convinced, allow the expectant mother to be taken to term, with delivery of a viable infant, without fear of convulsions. It has been shown in other clinics that eclampsia is fifty times more common in the diabetic than in the rest of the pregnant population. In the young severe diabetic patient it has yet to be proved that these three nutrients will prevent convulsions. On the other hand, the full story of diabetes in relation to B_6 is still unfolding. There is laboratory evidence, to be presented in Chapter 11, to indicate that B_6-deficient animals become diabetic.

The most difficult case I experienced in these 225 pregnant patients was that of S. S., twenty, in her first pregnancy. She was a severe diabetic. Hers was the only case of eclampsia that I observed, and her diabetes was, no doubt, a significant factor in it. When she arrived in my office, four months pregnant, on March 4, 1970, she had had diabetes for about two years and had taken the drug tolbutanide until it was replaced in February 1970 by twenty to thirty units of insulin daily.

Her family history was significant. Her mother had suffered severe edema with her first pregnancy and, more recently, had had edema of the hands, paresthesia of the hands, and painful menopausal arthritis of the hands and fingers. The recent conditions had all shown a remarkable response to pyridoxine. S. S.'s paternal grandfather, at seventy-five, had had an unusual stiffness and rheumatism, edema of the hands, and paresthesia; all had responded to pyridoxine.

These three individuals—S. S., her mother, her paternal grandfather—had lived in the same household for years and had eaten off the same table.

For about three years S. S. had been getting 50 milligrams of pyridoxine from a multivitamin capsule she took daily. On her first office visit for pregnancy I substituted a prenatal capsule and pyridoxine tablet that insured her 125 milligrams of B_6 daily.

But her edema, in the hands, became progressively more apparent. By July her rings had to be removed; elastic stockings were used to control the edema in her feet and ankles. Increasing pyridoxine to 425 milligrams daily helped but little. At the end of the month, on July 30, S. S. went to the hospital in active labor, with high blood pressure at 144/100 and 4-plus albumin in her urine. Edema, hypertension, albuminuria—she had all the signs of toxemia. Yet, although a diabetic, her blood sugar the next morning was almost normal at 77 milligrams percent, while her blood pressure had jumped to 160/100. She was then given 100 milligrams of pyridoxine, *but no insulin.*

Two serious complications presented themselves. The fetus was large, which is common with diabetic mothers, and it was in a breech position. I took her to the operating room to perform a Caesarean section. A ten-pound, seven-and-one-half-ounce male infant was delivered; he was normal and cried spontaneously. Before closing the incisions I injected oxytocin into the uterus. Oxytocin, a very strong hormone of the posterior pituitary gland, increases the contractions of the uterus during childbirth and helps prevent, or stop, bleeding afterward.

On the operating table she had 50 c.c. of lactated Ringer's solution intravenously while awaiting a pint of blood. The Ringer's solution contained calcium, sodium, and potassium—*but none of the solutions she received contained any magnesium.*

By 11 o'clock that morning the patient was awake and talked to the recovery-room nurse. All seemed to be going fine. Thirty minutes later, however, she went into a *grand mal* convulsion. Immediately she was injected with sodium phenobarbital and sodium dilantin to relax her, followed by similar doses thirty minutes later.

An hour after her last injection she had another *grand mal* convulsive seizure; her blood pressure was extremely high, and her blood sugar level was far above normal. One hour after the second seizure she was awake and coherent and apparently well, and her blood pressure had dropped to a normal range.

But by 4:00 P.M. her blood sugar had soared, and subsequently she was given ten units of insulin. Thirty minutes later she went into violent *grand mal* convulsions that continued until a large dose of magnesium sulfate was given. The convulsions then ceased. The patient went to sleep. (During the time of her convulsions, on the advice of a consulting physician I had also given her reserpine. Reserpine is a crystalline alkaloid used in treating hypertension. It is the only occasion on which I have used an antihypertensive agent in my pregnant patients.) Thereafter magnesium sulfate and reserpine were given for the next twenty-four hours, but it is doubtful that the reserpine had anything to do with relief from convulsions. A few days later, both mother and child were discharged from the hospital in good condition. (A detailed account of this case is presented in the Appendix.)

Like any case from which a physician learns a great deal, there were both negative and positive features. Certainly pyridoxine, given at the dosage of 425 milligrams daily, had not prevented convulsions, edema in the feet, hypertension, albuminuria, or an excessive birth weight of the baby of more than ten pounds. Presumably the diabetic status of the patient was a great factor. Yet on the positive side, both mother and infant survived to term, the mother went through twelve hours of labor climaxed by the stress of a Caesarean section—a major operation—before beginning convulsions, and the mother experienced no neuropathies in the prenatal period.

Without doubt the convulsions were finally halted in this case by the magnesium sulfate. Persons familiar with the drug reserpine might suggest that its action was delayed enough to have had little or no effect on the outcome. Nor were the powerful central nervous-system depressants—6 grains of sodium phenobarbital, 4½ grains of sodium dilantin, and 75 milligrams of meperidine—sufficient to stop convulsions during the eight hours between onset and final relief, which came immediately after administering magnesium sulfate. *Biochemists have proved that pyridoxine and magnesium are co-factors in several important enzymatic reactions in the human being, and there may have been some relationship in this case.* Magnesium sulfate has been used for decades in treating the convulsions of eclampsia. My father, a horse-and-buggy doctor, and many other older practitioners used Epsom salts—magnesium sulfate—as the standard treatment for toxemia, thinking the bowel action caused by cathartic medication helped the patient; but it seems more logical to think that the needed magnesium did the good.

Beginning with the fourth month of pregnancy in this diabetic patient, 125 milligrams of pyridoxine were given daily, along with 100 milligrams of magnesium oxide and 1 milligram of magnesium sulfate. But convulsions were halted only when a far greater amount of magnesium sulfate was used—1,250 milligrams injected into the vein and 1,000 milligrams into the muscle. *And it is to be emphasized that this woman had her worst convulsions after receivin ten units of regular insulin.*

My observations have led me to conclude that there are six factors contributing to convulsions in a pregnant woman. They are:

1. B_6 deficiency or increased need for B_6 as a result of the high estrogen balance during pregnancy, which becomes great during the last trimester.

2. Edema because of B_6 deficiency.

3. Increasing magnesium deficit associated with nausea and vomiting.

4. Malnutrition and poor intake are made worse if the patient is given great quantities of milk; the oversupply of calcium adds to the imbalance. Milk is a poor source for magnesium and B_6.

5. Lactation, which actually begins a few hours before the infant is born, makes the calcium-magnesium imbalance more acute.

6. If the patient has diabetes, her insulin injections provide a driving force that further changes the intracellular electrolyte balance, at the expense of magnesium. Magnesium is in close association with phosphorus in the intracellular exchanges, and B_6 is important as a co-factor with magnesium in phosphorilation. It appears clear to me that insulin, coupled with electrolyte imbalance, triggers convulsions in the eclamptic patient. The eclamptic patient is, in a sense, hypersensitive to insulin. (Other evidence to support this conclusion will be presented in Chapter 9.)

It must be emphasized again that diet was not changed in these patients, except in the few instances I have pointed out, and there was no restriction of salt intake at any time, whether there was edema or not. It has not been my experience that edema was caused by salt intake. Edema was, in nearly all cases, reduced by pyridoxine taken in adequate therapeutic amounts. Usually a reduction of swelling in the hands and feet of pregnant women could be seen within seventy-two hours. Weight loss might continue for ten days to two weeks, or the weight might remain stationary and with no further gain for the following two weeks.

Except for the injections of reserpine at the suggestion of a consulting colleague in the case of eclampsia just described, no antihypertensive drug was given during this ten-year period in which I delivered more than 225 babies. Yet five different patients, from fifteen to twenty-one years of age, which is a prime age group for eclampsia, recorded blood pressures of 170/110, 170/118, 180/120, 150/90, and 180/120 while in the hospital for delivery. The only therapeutic treatment they received was pyridoxine supplemented by near-minimal amounts of other vitamins and minerals. This strongly suggests that lowering the blood pressure with antihypertensive drugs is not essential for prevention of convulsions, as has been widely believed. Ultimately there seemed to be no risk involved in not using antihypertensive agents; also, it has never been suggested that hypertension in the mother causes hypertension in the fetus.

From these limited observations I would suggest that we might hereafter separate the three signs of eclampsia—temporarily fixed hypertension, edema, and convulsions. If pyridoxine can eliminate edema and assist in halting convulsions—as I believe it will—it is quite possible that the remaining sign, hypertension, could be more easily controlled, and overall mortality of eclampsia could be reduced, if not prevented. It is to be emphasized that the full role of large therapeutic doses of pyridoxine and magnesium in the prenatal period is just beginning to unfold. More investigations in large clinics are needed.

In evaluating the fluctuating edema of the hands during pregnancy, as well as in the premenstrual period and as a complication of menopausal arthritis, it seems certain that vitamin B₆ deficiency is in some way complicated by an imbalance of steroids, which is manifested by edema. As mentioned previously, there is laboratory evidence that estrogen, a female hormone, is intimately associated with B$_6$ metabolism. A sufficient amount of B$_6$ must be present for proper metabolism of estrogen; otherwise, the patient apparently becomes toxic from estrogen. This was covered in more detail in the chapter on carpal tunnel syndrome.

One other patient must be briefly mentioned in this discussion of eclampsia. R. Y. was a seventeen-year-old Afro-American who was thought to have eclampsia on September 30, 1967. She suffered a sudden onset of *grand mal* convulsions. These followed a ten-pound weight gain the previous week, which had been associated with edema, severe headaches, and a blood pressure reading of 170/100. At the time of convulsions, four weeks before she went into delivery, she was given 1,950 milligrams of pyridoxine over a seventy-hour period and was told to take 200 milligrams of pyridoxine daily thereafter until the birth of the baby.

She recovered from the convulsions, but on admission to the hospital twenty-eight days after her convulsive seizures her blood pressure was up to 166/110, and at the height of labor it reached a high of 182/120. Nonetheless, the baby, apparently healthy, was born October 28 without complications except that of severe hypertension in the mother.

However, two and one half years later the same patient R. Y. entered the hospital emergency room convulsing for the second time in life, and this time she was not pregnant. The diagnosis was epilepsy, and, based on this, it must be assumed that the accurate prenatal diagnosis was toxemia of pregnancy with complications of epilepsy rather than eclampsia. Whether or not pyridoxine had any effect on preventing convulsions at the time of labor must remain a matter of conjecture. It should be emphasized that when the patient returned with epileptic seizures two and a half years after the pregnancy, she was taking birth-control pills that contained estrogen and she was not taking B$_6$. For several years it has been known that epileptics do not tolerate contraceptive pills. Here again is clinical evidence of an estrogen–B$_6$ relationship in a patient with epilepsy.

A classic case of a patient who might be considered pre-eclamptic is that of V. M., twenty-four, pregnant for the first time. But edema was controlled and eclampsia was very likely prevented by a combination of B$_6$, magnesium, and potassium therapy. Her case sums up, in one patient, what I have learned with these 225 pregnant patients. (Her case is given in detail in the Appendix.)

She worked in a chicken-processing plant, exercising her hands constantly as she handled 5,000 chickens daily. When I first examined her she was two months pregnant, and I prescribed a total of 125 milligrams of pyridoxine daily, along with her prenatal capsule. Two months later she developed pain and swelling in her left hand, which grew worse. I diagnosed it as carpal tunnel syndrome and increased her pyridoxine to 325 milligrams daily and suggested she continue working. Within three days the left hand seemed normal and she had perfect flexion.

Continuing her 325-milligram dosage another month, she had no swelling in her hands or feet, but she did have very slight numbness in the tips of some of her fingers on the left hand. As she was planning to quit work, because of her general discomfort, I reduced her B$_6$ dosage to 125 milligrams daily, since she had no edema or complaints in her hands.

But in her ninth month she developed edema of the feet but no numbness or tingling in the hands. Other signs were alarming, enough to give an obstetrician gray hair overnight. Her blood pressure shot up extremely high, and she had a small amount of albumin in her urine. She had toxemia and was, possibly, a step away from convulsions, or eclampsia.

I thought convulsions could be headed off. I hiked her pyridoxine back up to 325 milligrams and now added large doses of magnesium and potassium. Within two weeks the edema was reduced. Twenty-two days after this additional therapy, she went into labor. She still had high blood pressure and albuminuria, *but there was absolutely no edema in her hands or feet. One could see the outline of every tendon on the back of her hands and the top of her feet.*

A healthy seven-pound, two-and-one-half-ounce female baby was born. Thirty-six hours after giving birth, mother and child were discharged from the hospital without complications. V. M. was never given a diuretic or an antihypertensive drug. She had been given only one sedative, and of course oxytocin and ergonovine were not used. She had had toxemia and still had hypertension and albuminuria at the time of birth. In the prenatal period she had had all of the signs and symptoms of the carpal tunnel syndrome associated with pregnancy. Yet she had not convulsed. Why? *Because, in my opinion, the combination of B_6 and magnesium had prevented eclampsia. Pyridoxine had relieved the carpal tunnel syndrome within three days, and it had done even more, in the body where we could not see.*

Based on my treatment of 225 pregnant women who received increased amounts of pyridoxine, at least seventeen conclusions were reached.

1. One may safely give 50 to 450 milligrams of pyridoxine daily and up to 1,000 milligrams daily for short intervals of three to five days during hospital confinement for delivery.

2. Edema of pregnancy was controlled or prevented by 50 to 450 milligrams daily in all but six patients. It was a conclusion that these six required additional B complex by injection or else that they were not absorbing their B_6 properly when it was taken by mouth.

3. Paresthesia of the hands and fingers, characterized by numbness, tingling, and loss of sensation in the fingertips, was relieved by 50 to 450 milligrams daily.

4. Dropping of objects, such as teacups and dinner plates, was relieved by 50 to 450 milligrams daily. This was interpreted as an improvement in hand grip as well as finger flexion and coordination.

5. Occasional nocturnal paralysis of an arm and hand following sleep was relieved by pyridoxine.

6. Salt restriction was unnecessary for prevention of edema when pyridoxine was given in therapeutic amounts.

7. Diuretic drugs were not necessary for treatment of any of the 225 pregnant women.

8. In spite of severe hypertension in patients with toxemia, with one exception, antihypertensive drugs were not used and seemed unnecessary and unassociated with prevention of convulsions.

9. There was the condition of diabetes mellitus in the only patient who did convulse within twenty-four hours of delivery.

10. Severe muscle spasms of the legs and feet of pregnant women were improved or completely relieved by 50 to 450 milligrams of pyridoxine daily.

11. Giving therapeutic doses of pyridoxine to pregnant women did not cause an increased need for vitamin B$_6$ in their infants.

12. There were associated epileptic-type convulsive seizures in one adult in this series, who also had toxemia. The convulsions apparently responded to pyridoxine.

13. Therapeutic doses of the two co-factors, pyridoxine and magnesium, were indicated for prevention of convulsions in patients with toxemia of pregnancy and treatment of convulsions of eclampsia.

14. Pain in the interphalangeal joints of the fingers was relieved when 50 to 450 milligrams of pyridoxine were given daily.

15. Pregnant women with extensive edema of the hands, feet, and legs lost from ten to fifteen pounds of weight within two weeks when given 50 to 450 milligrams of pyridoxine daily.

16. Induction of labor was not necessary, and patients were allowed to go to term delivery in all cases, regardless of appearance of toxemia.

17. It appears that the diabetic pregnant patient with eclampsia and with an electrolyte imbalance is hypersensitive to insulin and that insulin triggers convulsions.

These conclusions indicate that *all* pregnant women should have at least 50 milligrams of B$_6$ as a supplement throughout their pregnancies, and many of them will require considerably more than that. *All* pregnant women should also receive at least 500 milligrams of magnesium daily, and with the appearance of the signs of toxemia the magnesium should be increased to 1,000 milligrams daily.

Life Before, and After, Birth | 8

While a pregnant woman is suffering from B_6 deficiency and is being treated for it, what is happening to her unborn baby? What happens to these babies when they become children? What is the role of B_6 in the human being during that slow development into adulthood?

Fortunately, we do have a body of clinical data that provides us with many of the answers to these questions. During my investigations of B_6 during pregnancy I necessarily observed the babies as well as their mothers. In the process I accumulated detailed information that indicates a vital role for B_6 in the fetus as well as following birth.

Since 1961 I have delivered about 225 babies of mothers who were given from 50 to 450 milligrams of B_6 daily during pregnancy. Of these, only two infants showed evidence of an increased need for B_6 after birth, and they will be discussed in detail subsequently. This series included six sets of twins, plus breech deliveries, those with birth weights of less than five pounds, and other unrelated complications of pregnancy. As stated in the preceding chapter, maternal mortality was 0. Infant mortality was less than 2 percent.

There were five infants with known birth defects. One of them had coarctation of the aorta (stricture reducing the normal volume of the aorta), one had a supernumerary digital appendage on each hand (extra fingers), one had cleft lip, another was premature and had convulsions in an incubator soon after birth (which I will be discussing in this chapter), and another gave evidence of mental retardation with associated convulsions at eight months of age. The mother who gave birth to the infant with coarctation of the aorta was receiving 50 milligrams of pyridoxine daily when pregnancy began. The mother of the baby with the cleft lip got no pyridoxine supplements until the last trimester of pregnancy.

One result of B_6 therapy during pregnancy has been a quite unusual effect on some of the babies. It has happened a number of times, but the case of J. W., thirty-two, very obese, and in her ninth pregnancy, is a classic one. On April 18, 1968, approximately one month before giving birth, she walked barefoot into my office. It was her first trip to the doctor and her husband was in jail. She had massive edema of the hands, feet, and legs. She was so swollen that she couldn't wear shoes. She also complained of severe headache, blurred vision, severe foot and leg cramps, and severe paresthesia of the hands that she described as numbness and tingling. She was placed on 300 milligrams of pyridoxine daily for the next five weeks, with no other medication or supplement. Her headaches subsided, her hands and feet became wrinkled, the paresthesia subsided in her hands, the muscle cramps of the feet and legs vanished, and when she entered the hospital on May 19, ready to give birth, she was wearing a ring on the same finger she had worn it before she became pregnant. Although her blood pressure was high—at 180/100—her urine was negative for albumin and sugar, and she delivered a nine-pound, three-ounce infant male who cried spontaneously.

J. W.'s history, as we have seen in Chapter 7, has been duplicated by others, with only the details varying. With her infant son, however, something new and very striking entered the picture.

At birth the infant exhibited unusual wrinkling of the skin on the hands, feet, legs, arms, and trunk of his body. This is not normally seen. His skin was so wrinkled that it resembled that of a person who has been bathing in a swimming pool for several hours.

This phenomenon puzzled me at first. There seemed to be something different about the subcutaneous water deposits in the infant. In order to have a definite, objective record of the child I made motion pictures of him approximately twenty-four hours after birth.

The cause of this unusual wrinkling did not become clear until some time afterward, when I had delivered a number of babies of mothers who had had extensive edema in the last month of pregnancy. Eventually a pattern formed. These mothers had extensive edema. Their treatment began in the final month of pregnancy with large doses of pyridoxine. At parturition they gave birth to infants with this unusual wrinkling of skin. I soon had motion pictures of three such infants who clearly demonstrated that their skin was loose, wrinkled and totally devoid of that puffy or edematous appearance of many newborn babies.

At first I feared that large doses of pyridoxine had, in some way, dehydrated the fetus. Then as I thought my way through the unseen process, logically from cause to effect, a quite different procedure seemed likely. If the mother had been extremely edematous in that last month, I realized, then the fetus surely had not been exempt from the condition. Edema in the fetus must have accompanied edema in the mother. Thus, when vitamin B₆ had relieved edema in the mother, it must also have relieved edema in the fetus *in utero*. At parturition, both mother and baby had exhibited wrinkling skin; the mother's skin had previously been puffy and tight. There was an excellent chance that edema had subsided in the fetus the same time as it had in the mother.

One of these infants did not urinate for twenty-four hours following birth, and there was very little weight loss after birth. All of these three infants had less than the usual loss of weight during their first seventy-two hours in the world, a time when weight loss is predictable. This, it seemed to me, indicated that the babies had no excess fluid they needed to lose; the pyridoxine had already taken care of that.

When pyridoxine was given the mothers early in pregnancy, this unusual wrinkling of the skin was not apparent in their babies. Furthermore, the babies of these women were neither puffy nor edematous when they were delivered. A striking characteristic of several babies I have delivered is that they lost little or no weight in the hospital after birth. All of these features, added together, in my opinion, pay tribute to the therapeutic value of pyridoxine to the fetus as well as the mother. The general rule, all over the United States, is that babies lose several ounces of weight following delivery, some more than others. This suggests that such is true because the average fetus has prenatal edema, as its mother does, and the excess fluid is lost after birth. But with B_6 actively preventing or eliminating the excess fluids *in utero* these babies have proved themselves an exception to the general rule in this country and perhaps in many other countries. Over and over I have observed this phenomenon, and I am positive that vitamin B_6 is important in prevention of edema in the fetus.

Of the 225 babies delivered, only two of them showed an increased need for vitamin B_6, as I was able to determine it. Both of these infants were born of mothers who had marked edema of pregnancy; one of the mothers had toxemia.

One of the infants, D. S., was born a fraternal twin of a mother who in a previous pregnancy had demonstrated a high degree of edema that responded to pyridoxine, plus B-complex injections. On admission to the hospital, on November 30, 1965, when D. S. was born, the mother had albumin in the urine (1-plus), and her blood pressure ranged from 132/96 to 150/90.

D. S. did not develop normally. At eight months of age she could not lift her head from a pillow. She would not hold a bottle or reach for it if it were beside her, and the mother had to hold the infant in her lap to feed the baby. In the bassinet the baby would attempt little movement and lay on her back with no apparent desire to try to crawl. *It was impossible to get her to grasp and hold a baby rattle, spoon, or any other object.* By this time a pattern had been established; she developed convulsions when she experienced any elevation of temperature.

She was given pyridoxine by mouth (12 milligrams daily). Within one week D. S. was attempting to crawl about her bassinet, playing, clutching and shaking her baby rattle vigorously and with good coordination, and she held her bottle while drinking her milk. It was a striking change.

Subsequently, as a child her case was diagnosed as epilepsy, and she was treated with pyridoxine (50 milligrams daily) and dilantin

(125 milligrams twice daily), a drug used in treating epileptic attacks. She received nothing else. At six years of age she had a convulsive seizure. A few minutes later a blood-sugar determination revealed her glucose blood level to be 80 milligrams percent— apparently normal. In order to check her more thoroughly, the following day a six-hour glucose tolerance test was done, during which the blood sugar ranged from a fasting level of 81 milligrams percent up to a high of 188 milligrams percent at the one-half-hour mark and down to a low of 78 milligrams percent at six hours. Although there was a rather high and low excursion it was within the limits of what is generally considered normal; a possible explanation for the quite high one-half-hour reading could be that the laboratory gave her 100 grams of dextrose instead of the 50 grams usually recommended for one of her age and weight. The test had, however, ruled out the possibility that her epileptic seizures were associated with abnormally low blood sugar in this particular individual. Her glucose tolerance test gave these results:

Fasting	½ Hour	1 Hour	2 Hours	3 Hours	4 Hours	5 Hours	6 Hours
81 mg. %	188	118	102	90	84	80	78

At age six D. S. was a rather pretty little girl. Although she had to have special education in school, she could talk, liked to draw pictures with coloring pencils, had a nice smile, and seemed happy enough.

T. G., the second infant who required an increased amount of B₆, was born prematurely and had convulsions in an incubator.

But first let us examine the infant T. G.'s prenatal history. His mother was nineteen years old and in her first pregnancy when she was first observed on October 12, 1963. She was given a multi-vitamin-mineral capsule (twice daily) that contained nine vitamins and six minerals, including 10 milligrams of pyridoxine, 830 milligrams of calcium carbonate, and only 1 milligram of magnesium sulfate. Two months later, on December 12, I added 50 milligrams of pyridoxine to this supplementation.

The mother seemed to be doing well until, on January 12, 1964, she discontinued taking pyridoxine, of her own accord. Thirty days later she developed toxemia of pregnancy, with extensive edema of the hands and feet. When pyridoxine was again given (100 milli-grams daily) along with the same multivitamin-mineral capsules, the edema subsided. But her blood pressure remained high; at the time of delivery it was 182/120. There were no complications, nor were forceps used in the delivery on April 14, 1964.

The baby, T. G., weighed three pounds, fourteen ounces, which classified him as premature, and he was placed in an incubator. *Eighty-one hours after birth, he began to have convulsions in the incubator.* Realizing that pyridoxine had been essential in prevent-ing convulsions in infants as early as the nineteen fifties, when the B_6-deficient commercial baby formula had been in use, I admin-istered 25 milligrams of pyridoxine by intramuscular injection. The convulsions promptly ceased. Forty minutes later, however, con-vulsions recurred and persisted for the next thirteen hours. The child had two more injections of pyridoxine (25 milligrams each) during the hospital stay, after all convulsions had ended. Once the convulsions ceased, the remaining hospital stay went smoothly for both mother and child.

Three weeks after birth the parents and infant T. G. moved to Fort Worth, Texas, where the boy remained until after he had started school. In December 1966, when he was two years old, T. G. was hospitalized for what was described as a "blackout." It was diagnosed as hypoglycemia, or low blood sugar, but he was placed on no special diet.

Almost one year later, on November 24, 1967, when he was three and a half years old and weighed thirty-five and a half pounds, he awoke apparently well but went back to sleep soon afterward. Offered food, he refused to eat, although he did take fluids. His mother then noted that he was staring blankly and seemed to be unaware of his surroundings. He began screaming and was still screaming when seen by the pediatrician. There was no vomiting, no diarrhea, no actual convulsions in rigidity. Except for the pre-vious year, he had been hospitalized one other time, for pneumonia; he had no known allergies and there was no history of hypoglycemia or epilepsy in the family that his parents knew of.

On admission to the hospital in Fort Worth, his urine albumin was 2-plus, with a 3-plus acetone, and his blood sugar was recorded as 30 milligrams percent—extremely low. The acetone reading indicated he was incompletely metabolizing his sugar. Albuminuria meant he was spilling part of life's vital protein in the kidney. When he was tested for a possible intracranial mass, which is a standard pediatric procedure in such cases, his chest and skull X rays were negative and normal, ruling out organic disease in those areas. His red blood count, cholesterol (145 milligrams percent), and urea nitrogen (18 milligrams percent) were all within normal ranges. An EEG, or electroencephalogram, was taken of his brain tracings. It proved to be abnormal, in the words of the attending physician, "consistent with and suggestive of a generalized paroxysmal convulsive disorder."

Next he was given a five-hour glucose tolerance test. By then it was nearly three days following the onset of symptoms. No sugar or acetone turned up in the urine at any point. His fasting level was 89 milligrams percent; the highest level was 145 and the lowest, at four hours, 73, which was 16 points below his fasting level. At no point during the test did he go as low as his admitting blood-sugar level of 30. No dietary change was suggested by the attending physician.

Learning from a relative that T. G. was again having seizures at age three, I suggested to the relative that it might be best that the boy resume taking pyridoxine. He was thereafter given 25 milligrams daily for the next year and then 50 milligrams daily for the next four years. During this period he had no more convulsive seizures or "blackouts."

T. G. began the first grade of school in Fort Worth. Shortly afterward his parents divorced. The child was brought back to Mt. Pleasant in November 1970. He became withdrawn, uncommunicative with his teacher, "seemed as if he were in a shell," and failed to pass his grade that year. His mother attributed this to difficult psychological adjustments, which seemed to be a reasonable possibility. This background became obvious to me in March 1972, when the mother sought medical attention for his problems. During the intervening years since his birth I had seen him on one occasion, for a cold, and of course was not aware of many of the details I have set forth here until March when I talked with his mother.

Following the examination, I sent the child to a laboratory for a six-hour glucose tolerance test on March 22, 1972, which gave these results:

Fasting	½ Hour	1 Hour	2 Hours	3 Hours	4 Hours	5 Hours	6 Hours
90 mg. %	80	75	70	45	70	75	70

This was interpreted as a "flat" sugar tolerance curve, except for a low of 45. He does not seem to have had any unusual reaction during the test; afterward he played sandlot baseball with the neighborhood children for two hours before eating supper. Prior to the six-hour glucose tolerance test he had not been on any kind of diet; he had eaten what he wanted, including ice cream, candy, and desserts at the school cafeteria.

On the basis of the test and his history I diagnosed him as a reactive hypoglycemic and on March 22 placed him on a high-protein, medium-fat, low-carbohydrate diet, which he tolerated well. In the event it may not be well understood by non-doctors, the hypoglycemic—the patient suffering from low blood sugar—has a problem in the metabolism of sugar and other refined carbohydrates. This means he must sharply curtail his intake of sugar and refined carbohydrates, as paradoxical as it may seem. Current thought is that heavy loads of sugar released into the bloodstream cause the pancreas to overreact and put too much insulin into the blood. It appears that the imbalance of insulin brings the blood sugar level too far down in these patients. Therefore, protein, especially, and fats are used to maintain a stable supply of glucose in the blood.

Following the administration of the six-hour glucose tolerance test, I reviewed T. G.'s records, including those of the initial convulsions in the incubator. As was the accepted custom of caring for premature infants, one-fourth ounce of 5 percent glucose was fed the infant at two-hour intervals for seven feedings, beginning twenty-eight hours after birth. The convulsions did not begin until eighty-one hours after birth. It seems possible that if the infant had a convulsion from reactive hypoglycemia at age three, then he could also have had initial convulsions from glucose intolerance. At the 1964 International Symposium on B_6 it was pointed out that there is low blood glucose, or sugar, and low glucose tolerance in B_6 deficiency, resulting in a sensitivity to insulin; others have reported the fasting blood sugar level, in B_6 deficiency, as within the normal range, although B_6 has been shown to be a factor in the forming of more liver glycogen (a sugar stored in the liver), and its longer retention, than is true of B_6-deficient animals.[1,2]

Following the glucose feedings he received as an infant, T. G. was given a high-protein milk formula that is usually given premature infants. A conclusion might be drawn that pyridoxine probably was of some benefit in controlling convulsions associated with reactive hypoglycemia.

In the kind of follow-up report that causes doctors to beam on getting, T. G.'s mother called me on April 29, 1972, the month after his glucose tolerance test, to inform me that her son "really is doing good since you put him on the diet." This withdrawn child was not the same, she said. "I am really proud of his diet. Before the diet he sat around like he had no energy. His teacher said he is so different at school. The teacher says she has noticed considerable change; she even had to scold him a couple of times because he was 'picking' at other children, something he has never done in the past." Now he had the energy to misbehave occasionally!

A few days later I telephoned his teacher for confirmation. Mrs. Iona Carpenter, a highly skilled professional with master's degrees in elementary education and psychology of the exceptional child, had over the past seven years taught reading and spelling to about two hundred children who had a specific language disability (dyslexia).

"Before beginning treatment with the special [high-protein, low-carbohydrate] diet," said Mrs. Carpenter, "T. G. would sit in his seat withdrawn from all around him, as if he were dreaming all by himself. He had no interest in school work, and it was difficult to hold his attention. He frowned all the time. His movements were slow, coordination was poor, and he seemed to have little energy. He walked slowly and seemed to be slow in motion. I had to stand in the door to wait for him to arrive to begin nearly every class."

After he had started the high-protein, low-carbohydrate diet, Mrs. Carpenter noted a sharp, specific change in his behavior. "Now he pays attention to what he is being told, and he arrives at his class on time. Coordination in his movements has improved and he walks faster. There has been a definite improvement in his work habits. His reading has improved, and he has asked for a new reader to take home for practice reading. His mood has changed, and he talks to children around him. He laughs now, whereas before he appeared as if he didn't really care about life."

Some very important insights were provided by the T. G. case. Born prematurely of a mother suffering from toxemia of pregnancy —including edema of pregnancy that responded to pyridoxine before his birth—T. G. showed some response to B_6 in the incubator after he began convulsing. At the age of three he convulsed again. Between the ages of three and eight he received from 25 to 50 milligrams of pyridoxine daily—and had no convulsions or "black-outs" thereafter, even though he survived on a high-carbohydrate diet that included candies, cookies, carbonated drinks, and ice cream almost daily.

The most important factor is that a dietary imbalance caused much of his difficulty. He either had an intolerance to a diet high in carbohydrates or else he needed the high-protein diet to supply something he wasn't getting. He also needed more pyridoxine than his peers. The results of a proper diet were little short of incredible. Dietary improvement changed his mood—from one of frustration and despair to one of accomplishment, happiness, and a zest for life.

This finding is not unique to my experience but only adds support to findings of many medical colleagues who have been searching for the proper concept of hypoglycemia (low blood sugar), dyslexia, and depressive psychosis. It is certain that this child, T. G., had a failure in carbohydrate metabolism, that it probably caused convulsions in the incubator when he received a dilute glucose formula, and that he very likely needed a high-protein, low-carbohydrate diet supported by an increased amount of pyridoxine, beginning with the first day of his life.

Medical people are still actively discussing the causes of mental retardation, prematurity, low birth weights, hypoglycemia, and psychoses associated with malnutrition. It is well accepted, however, that premature infants often have immature systems of enzymes and that specific food antagonists, such as galactose and leucine, are capable of triggering or precipitating convulsive seizures in certain individuals.

It is also of some significance that persons on high-protein diets automatically need more B_6—for B_6 is the "protein vitamin" that is needed to help utilize protein. For this reason, if for no other, *all hypoglycemics should receive B_6 supplements, in addition to their special diets.*

Except for the two children mentioned in this chapter, the infants that I delivered of mothers on B_6 appear to be normal or better than normal in observable ways. They grew normally, showed no dependency on B_6, and are now doing successful work in grade school or kindergarten. Those who are not yet old enough for kindergarten appear bright and active. But a few infants, such as T. G. and D. S., are born with an *increased need* for B_6.

In medical language, those persons who have a prolonged requirement for above-normal levels of pyridoxine to control symptoms are classified as "B_6-dependent." This does not refer at all to such things as addiction or "habit." For the clarification of the non-doctor, "B_6-dependent" means merely that continued supplementation of vitamin B_6 is necessary for these persons whose needs are greater than the normal person. The term "B_6 dependency" was introduced in 1954 by Drs. Andrew D. Hunt, Jr., Joseph Stokes, Jr., Wallace W. McCrory, and H. H. Stroud. They have indicated that some infants are dependent on large doses of B_6 for survival. In the first case they reported that the mother had been given pyridoxine in the second, third, fourth, and fifth months of pregnancy, but apparently she was not given pyridoxine in the sixth, seventh, eighth, and ninth months. They speculated that the high dosages of pyridoxine during these early months had caused an inborn metabolic error.[3] However, my work subsequently, in which mothers were given pyridoxine in the late as well as the early months of pregnancy, has definitely shown that large doses of B_6 given to the pregnant mother do not cause such an inborn error of metabolism.

These two patients, D. S. and T. G., appear to be what Hunt *et al.* referred to as B_6-dependent children. Other observers, including Dr. David B. Coursin, have found that some children require additional amounts of pyridoxine daily in order to prevent convulsive seizures. By the time this condition is discovered and analyzed properly, some children are found to be mentally retarded. Myelinization of the nerves is not complete until near the end of the first year of life. In South America and Africa epidemiologists have shown that mental retardation was permanent in starving infants who did not have adequate vitamins, minerals, and protein during the first year of life.

Animal experiments have shown that birth defects are very striking in association with B_6-deficient diets. Such diets may cause irreversible damage. Reports from clinics and laboratories have revealed a definite relationship between increased need for B_6 and mental retardation.[4]

The picture, however, is far, far from being complete. Mysteries abound in the story of B_6. Some of the more puzzling facets are to be found in how the vitamin deficiency affects the very young. Paul György has called attention to two particularly perplexing questions: Why is it that in young animals and infants B_6 deficiency is manifested in convulsion, while in older subjects it is more often shown in anemia? And why are B_6-dependent convulsions more common in the female but B_6-dependent anemia more common in the male? Does the answer lead back to the interrelationship of the vitamin and hormones?[5]

Granted that B_6 deficiency in the fetus may cause birth defects and create problems for the infant after birth, including those involving B_6 dependency, what about the older child and the youth? Do any of them have medical problems related to insufficient B_6? Apparently B_6 needs do not show up dramatically until later years, but I have treated this sort of patient during teenage years.

One Sunday morning a cowboy's wife fell and fractured her ankle. I had just finished putting a plaster-of-Paris cast on her leg and ankle and was waiting for a post-reduction X-ray film to develop when her younger brother said to me, "Doctor, I can't get my ring off. My hands are swollen and they feel terrible, they hurt and tingle so much. I am going to have to cut my ring off."

The complaint sounded familiar but not from one so young as he. I asked him, "How old are you?"

"Seventeen."

I looked at his hands. "Let's see you flex the ends of your fingers to that crease there." I showed him how to do the QEW test.

At seventeen he was a strong, husky youngster weighing 173 pounds, but he couldn't press a single finger in either hand against the metacarpophalangeal crease!

"What else have you noticed?" I said.

"My stomach is swelled. It feels all blown up."

There were three holes in his belt, and he had buckled in the last hole to give him maximum circumference.

I didn't tell him what I thought was causing his problem in order not to prejudice him one way or the other. I wrote a prescription for fourteen pyridoxine tablets (50 milligrams each) and told him to take one a day, starting then, and return in thirteen days.

He did. Thirteen days later his ring, which he had feared he would have to cut off, slipped off his finger easily.

"My left hand doesn't tingle or hurt at all," he said. He pointed to the tip of the long finger of his right hand and explained, "I still have numbness of the tip of this finger."

When he stood up I could see that his belt was buckled in the first notch, the one for minimum circumference. He had taken it up two notches.

I had him run through the QEW test. He pressed every finger flat against the palmar interphalangeal crease.

When he returned a week later, his hands didn't hurt or tingle, and the numbness was gone in the long finger of his right hand. He had taught me that no age group is exempt from medical disorders requiring increased needs for vitamin B₆, from the time of gestation and birth all the way to that of old age.[6]

The Mystery of Diabetes | 9

Vitamin B_6 therapy may be a link in the prevention of diabetes as well as a number of other diseases.

In my own practice I have seen a relationship between the two that provides clinical clues in this direction. Many diabetics have turned up with signs and symptoms that, in other patients, were successfully treated with B_6. In turn the diabetic so suffering also benefited. Many patients with diabetes mellitus had disturbed tactile sensations in their fingers that responded to pyridoxine. Furthermore, I have noted that most elderly diabetics have edema in their hands and fingers, as well as neuritis and neuropathies in their hands and fingers. These conditions responded favorably to 50 milligrams of pyridoxine daily.

George S. Phalen, the surgeon cited in Chapter 4 as an authority on the carpal tunnel syndrome, found that 27 percent of his carpal tunnel syndrome patients either had diabetes or came from families with a history of diabetes. Thus, in examining a severe and serious syndrome of this nature, and which responds to B_6 therapy, one finds a significant statistical association between it and diabetes.

Furthermore, moving into the laboratory, animal experiments performed by the Japanese scientist Yakito Kotake and others have established a link between diabetes and vitamin B_6 deficiency. Tryptophan, an amino acid or protein, is eventually metabolized by the body into niacin, if it follows its normal pathway.[1] Vitamin B$_6$ is necessary for the degradation of tryptophan, as it is for every other amino acid studied. Xanthurenic acid is one of the metabolites of tryptophan; a high excretion of it in the urine indicates a disturbed metabolic process related to B$_6$ deficiency or malfunction. Kotake found xanthurenic acid to be present invariably in free form in the urine of diabetic patients.

Kotake and co-workers in Japan have also shown xanthurenic acid to be a cause of diabetes. Using a high fat diet in experimental animals, he found the diet increases the diabetogenic effects of xanthurenic acid by first reducing the glutathione content of the blood, binding insulin, and possibly leading to chronic diabetes as a result of the exhaustion of cells in the pancreas. (As a rule, diabetics eat more fat.) Of course, complete destruction of these particular cells in the pancreas cannot be reversed by pyridoxine, but Kotake has demonstrated that pyridoxine will prevent all manifestations of the diabetogenic effect of xanthurenic acid.

What, though, of the human patient, who is more complex and not as easily studied as the laboratory animal?

Obviously the relationship between the human diabetic and vitamin B$_6$ is necessarily going to be more difficult to show directly. But a case demonstrating the therapeutic effects of B$_6$ is that of L. B., a fifty-five-year-old cook who was first observed on February 15, 1967. He had probably cooked more meals for more persons in more cafés and restaurants than any cook in his part of the country, and his father before him had operated a café.

"I have cramps in my legs when I walk," said L. B. The cramps became worse when he walked as far as two city blocks. He had numbness and tingling in his hands and fingers. For the past twelve years he had been unable to wear his wedding ring because of the swelling in his hands. The sensation in his fingers had deteriorated to the point where he couldn't feel the weave in a tablecloth.

When I examined him, the pulsation of the dorsalis pedis arteries, those on the top of his feet, were barely perceptible because of arteriosclerosis. His hands were swollen, and as he attempted unsuccessfully to perform the QEW test he experienced pain in the interphalangeal joints of his fingers.

A laboratory workup revealed that he had 4-plus sugar in his urine; the urine was negative for albumin. Blood sugar was sufficiently high to classify him as a victim of diabetes mellitus.

Without initially changing the usual diet of his home and the café, an estimated 40 to 50 percent of which was fat, I put him on 50 milligrams of pyridoxine daily. Three weeks later, on March 8, the pain in his interphalangeal joints had subsided, edema was gone from the hands and fingers, and for the first time in twelve years L. B. was wearing his wedding ring. All his fingers could now be flexed properly for the QEW test.

And he volunteered this information: "Before I started taking the vitamin pill I couldn't feel the weave in a tablecloth. Now I can."

That day—March 8—he was given a 2,000-calorie diabetic diet, told to take one tolbutamide tablet daily, also for his diabetes, and to continue taking 50 milligrams of pyridoxine daily and indefinitely.

Well over a year later, on September 13, 1968, L. B. was sent to a Veterans Administration hospital. There, because of advanced arteriosclerosis, his terminal aorta and proximal iliac arteries were resected and replaced by a plastic arterial graft. Following this he returned to work as a cook.

During his seven weeks of treatment at the veterans hospital, he said, he received no pyridoxine supplements. When he was discharged he drove his automobile one hundred miles during the trip home. "My hands would go to sleep on the steering wheel," he said, "I'd have to drive with one hand and rub the other hand on my trousers."

When he got home he resumed taking pyridoxine, from 50 to 100 milligrams daily, and he could then clutch the steering wheel without any problems. When I talked with him by telephone on February 29, 1972, he was still taking 50 milligrams of pyridoxine a day, and the sensation in his hands was normal.

Because of my years of experience with this condition, I had anticipated his response to pyridoxine before treatment. I took motion pictures of his hands before treatment, then again afterward, in order to document objectively the reduction of edema and improved finger flexion.

The case of L. B. also brings to attention the dire predicament

of the blind diabetic patients who can no longer read Braille because of disturbed or lost tactile sensation in their fingertips. Much
has been written of these patients. L. B. was not a blind diabetic,
but he was a diabetic with disturbed tactile sensation. I have
treated a number of other diabetic patients with pyridoxine who
also reported a return of normal sensation to their fingertips following treatment. For the blind diabetic, the restoration of tactile
sensation in his fingertips is of vital significance. It restores an
additional link to the outside world as he perceives the written
word through his fingertips with the raised-dot coding of the Braille
system.

The medical complications that diabetics experience are usually
much more serious than those of the non-diabetic population. As
we have seen in Chapter 7, pregnant women who have diabetes
tend to have a much more difficult time of it than do others. This
pattern continues in non-pregnant diabetics as well.

In order to illustrate this difference, two cases will be presented
as a means of comparison. The first one, dealing with H. B., is of a
non-diabetic. The one that will follow hers is that of N. H., who
did have diabetes. The case of non-diabetic H. B. will serve to
demonstrate to us what may be expected of a "normal" patient
with this specific disorder as compared to a diabetic patient.

H. B., seventy-four, when seen on September 10, 1971, complained bitterly of painful shoulders, painful knees, and painful
hands and fingers. If she tried to pick up dishes she dropped and
broke them, she told me, and she couldn't sleep at night because
of pain from pressure on her shoulders. An examination revealed
her to have a pitting edema in her feet and ankles, as well as 50
percent loss of flexion in her fingers.

In order to explore her mental attitude toward her complaints
and to establish a time factor of eighteen days, I had her continue
to take the analgesics that she had been taking and to begin a
well-known tranquilizer three times daily. On her next visit, September 28, there was no change. She had tremulous, incomplete
flexion of her fingers, a 2-plus pitting edema of the feet and ankles,
and she was miserable.

I discontinued all medication she had been taking and put her
on 50 milligrams of pyridoxine daily.

Fourteen days later, on October 12, she reported, "I can lie with my hands in bed at night and they don't pain me like they did." By November 30 she had no edema in her feet and ankles and could flex all her fingers completely. The pain she had felt in her shoulders while lying in bed at night had subsided, and she could grip her dishes and cups without dropping and breaking them.

Her problems up to this point were much like those of many other patients I had treated. However, on February 29, 1972, H. B. developed an acute pain in her lower abdomen and began vomiting violently. For four days and nights she did not seek medical attention. Instead she took castor oil at home and by March 4 she had fecal vomiting. At this point she entered the hospital, where X rays revealed loops of small intestine distended with gas. A Levin tube, a nasal gastroduodenal catheter used in gastric and intestinal operations since 1921, was placed through the nose and into the stomach, and I prepared to explore the abdomen surgically.

It was 1:00 A.M. of March 5 when I completed the operation to remove a mass of adhesions that had caused a complete bowel obstruction. During the first twenty-four hours of her hospital stay H. B. was given 1,000 c.c. of a lactated Ringer's solution by clysis (in fat) and 2,000 c.c. of lactated Ringer's solution intravenously, as well as one pint of blood. Lactated Ringer's solution, also called the isotonic solution of three chlorides, contains sodium, potassium, and calcium. It is used in all forms of dehydration but particularly in cases in which a loss of gastrointestinal secretions has resulted from vomiting or diarrhea and when sodium, potassium, and calcium have been diminished. It is also used in acidosis or alkalosis for improvement of circulation and stimulation of renal activity.

The Levin tube was removed on March 6. During the operation and afterward there were no complications, and H. B. enjoyed an uneventful recuperation. She was discharged on March 23 in good condition and was subsequently seen in my office, still in good condition, on May 15.

Now H. B. did not have diabetes, but she had a long-standing need for vitamin B_6 and she had an acute bowel obstruction and had had no food in her stomach for seven days and nights. But H. B.'s case history gives us a "norm" against which to compare the case of N. H., which I will next present. N. H. had severe diabetes, an acute bowel obstruction. Initially, N. H. was treated much the same way as was H. B.; but N. H. developed convulsions.

N. H., fifty-eight, a seamstress, was seen first on January 9, 1967. For the six years preceding that day she had suffered with diabetes, for which she took thirty units of insulin daily.

"I am hurting all over," she said. "I can't sit down, lie down, or walk without pain in my arms, shoulders, knees, and ankles."

For the past six months she had been unable to hold cloth and pull a needle and thread through it; she didn't have enough grip in her hands. She couldn't make her thumbs touch the index fingers of either hand, and she couldn't touch the tips of her thumbs to the other fingers. Nor could she close her eyes and tell, from touch alone, what kind of cloth she had in her hands, for she had lost the sensation in the tips of her fingers.

Because she was a widow and now could not support herself, she had been receiving a welfare check and government commodities in order to get by.

I examined her. She had diffuse swelling in both hands; all of the interphalangeal joints were swollen and painful to both pressure and movement. She had a 50 percent loss of flexion at the interphalangeal joints of the fingers, and, to a lesser degree, *she was unable to extend her fingers completely.* (For those especially interested in hand function, note that extension at interphalangeal joints was also incomplete in many cases.) She had Heberden's nodes that were elevated, tender, and palpable near the interphalangeal joints of several fingers. She had what is known as "tennis elbow," a point tenderness near the elbow at the radiohumeral joints. Both knee joints had diffuse swelling and seemed to have fluid in them.

The lab data gave me a more precise picture of her condition. She had 4-plus sugar in the urine—high—but, with uric acid at 4.9 milligrams percent—normal. Hemoglobin was at 11.8 grams, good, with 5,000 white blood cells.

She was told to continue her usual diabetic diet and the thirty units of insulin daily. To this she was to add 50 milligrams of pyridoxine daily.

She returned on January 31 after having taken pyridoxine for three weeks. Overall she exhibited a marked improvement. Pain was remarkably reduced in the interphalangeal joints, and swelling was reduced in her hands and fingers. Although her Heberden's nodes were still obvious, they were much less painful. Her finger flexion was now complete; she passed the QEW test with ease by properly manipulating the tips of all fingers. Swelling had subsided in the knees. There was some residual pain in the elbows, but it, as well as that in the shoulders, was better. She could move her arms at the shoulders better.

Then she contributed this clincher: "I can close my eyes and feel cloth between my fingers and tell what kind of cloth I'm sewing on now."

By October 16 she had ten months of pyridoxine therapy behind her (50 milligrams daily). Now she could feel a lock of hair with her fingers, and for the first time she mentioned hand grip. "I didn't have enough strength in my hands before to pull a needle through cloth; now I can sew five hours a day." Before treatment her index and long fingers would lock in "trigger finger" fashion. Over the months the locking sign had disappeared.

N. H. was observed several times a year for the next five years. She remained on pyridoxine; she never once had a recurrence of the crippling condition she had in 1967. What was of perhaps greatest significance to her was that during this five-year period she had received no welfare checks and no government commodities. She had made her own living as a seamstress, now that she had recovered from her disability, and by January 1972 she was making a new dress each day.

At one point during this five-year period, however, N. H. entered a hospital in another city in an emergency situation. The attending physician subsequently sent me her records, which showed she had developed a bowel obstruction that was accompanied by severe abdominal cramps, nausea, and vomiting. A surgeon there, on opening her abdomen, found a section of gangrenous bowel, which included a large Meckel's diverticulum. (The diverticulum ilei is the persistent proximal end of the yolk stalk, which is the narrow, ductlike part of the yolk sac uniting it to the midgut.) This was resected successfully.

I will go into this 1969 hospitalization, although it was not under my observation, in some detail because it relates to a subsequent hospitalization, in 1972, that was under my supervision. During the first hour after admission in 1969 patient N. H. began some type of "convulsions with eyes rolled back and bouncing on the bed." Her blood sugar was a high 308 milligrams percent, and she was treated with intravenous fluids, barbiturates, and tranquilizers. The intravenous fluids included dextrose in water and a few bottles of lactated Ringer's solution.

On the eighth post-operative day she was still having considerable nausea and vomiting and, according to the nurses' notes, was "bouncing on the bed," meaning that she had had some type of convulsive seizure. *Prior to this she had received 1,000 c.c. of lactated Ringer's, to which was added 20 milliequivalents of potassium chloride and fifteen units of regular insulin.* During her hospital stay in the other city—February 23 to March 9—she received no vitamin therapy.

Unfortunately N. H. was one of the many victims of the influenza epidemic of the winter of 1972. Early in February she was hospitalized in another town because of a severe case of flu. I examined her on February 15, and although she was still in a very weakened condition, because of the flu, she was, in many ways, in good shape. She could flex all her fingers perfectly, scoring 100 percent on the QEW test. There was no evidence of swelling in her knees, and she had a full range of motion in the shoulders. Her Heberden's nodes were palpable but not tender. Sensation in the tips of her fingers was completely normal. She still took thirty units of insulin a day.

The next day, however, a near-tragic incident occurred that presented both positive and negative evidence regarding the therapeutic use of vitamin B₆ in the treatment of diabetes. She again developed a bowel obstruction, accompanied by violent abdominal cramps and incessant nausea and vomiting. Before she was hospitalized I noted that she had some involuntary tonic and clonic tremors in her legs that seemed to come and go. These are muscular contractions or spasms. That morning she had taken her insulin as usual but took no food all day because of vomiting. For this reason, on hospital admission she was given glucose intravenously. In her very weakened condition she soon went into a diabetic coma. She became lethargic, and had it not been for a mechanical respirator using oxygen her respirations would have stopped. It was an extremely critical time, with her life in the balance. She was given fifty units of regular insulin, with hourly blood sugars taken to monitor its impact. Eventually that day her blood sugar dipped to 52 milligrams, and an intravenous feeding of 10 percent dextrose was used to elevate her blood sugar, as seemed to be indicated.

After 7:00 P.M. on February 16, N. H.'s respirations were not in jeopardy, and her blood sugar, to a degree, stabilized around 200 milligrams percent—high for a normal person but not unusual for a diabetic.

However, from that point on, other events provided an unusual opportunity to study the relationship of electrolytes, vitamins, and fluid balance in a patient. The electrolytes are potassium, calcium, sodium, and magnesium. Throughout it must be remembered that N. H. was a severe diabetic patient, in the midst of an abdominal crisis, who had for five years shown a spectacular response to vitamin B_6 in relieving the crippling rheumatism in her hands.

Earlier that day, at 12:30 P.M., the laboratory determined from blood tests her serum electrolytes. These were: chloride, 103 milliequivalents per liter; potassium, 3.1 mEq/L; sodium, 142 mEq/L; calcium, 4.7 mEq/L; and blood sugar, 66 milligrams percent. A magnesium level was not determined because it was not a routine procedure in the hospital where I was working and the technician was unfamiliar with the technique for magnesium determination.

At about the same time the blood sample was taken, a continuous intravenous drip of lactated Ringer's solution was begun.*

By 7:00 P.M. on February 16, when N. H.'s respirations were

* The lactated Ringer's solution contained these electrolytes: sodium, 130 mEq/L; potassium, 4 mEq/L; calcium, 2.7 mEq/L; chloride, 109.7 mEq/L; and lactate, 27 mEq/L. To this was added 30 milliequivalents of potassium, plus the following vitamins: thiamine (vitamin B_1), 250 milligrams; ascorbic acid (vitamin C), 1,000 mg.; riboflavin (B_2), 50 mg.; niacinamide, 1,250 mg.; pyridoxine, 50 mg.; and sodium pantothenate, 500 mg.

satisfactory and her blood sugar seemed stabilized, she again began having involuntary tremors of the muscles of the legs. From time to time the nurse or a relative had to press firmly on her legs to halt these slight jerking movements. The patient became more nauseated, and she vomited violently until a Levin tube was placed through her nose and into her stomach to provide continuous stomach gavage.

Except for her intravenous drip she was receiving no fluids or food. Now her abdominal pain began to increase and she became hyperirritable. Even the slightest noises, such as a nurse opening the door, seemed to trigger new tremors of the arms and legs. She would roll back her eyes with a wide-open stare and literally shake the bed in a "bouncing type of convulsion." Throughout that night and the following day she went through a prolonged series of tremors, involving muscular spasms and contractions, every few minutes, almost in waves, that would end in mattress-shaking bouncing convulsions.

It was as terrifying an experience for observers as it would have been for the patient had she been conscious. What was mystifying was that one might possibly expect tremors or convulsions when the blood sugar level was 52 to 60 milligrams percent; yet this patient had had that level for only a few hours. At the time of frank convulsions the patient had a blood sugar of 276 milligrams percent.

Meanwhile, since the day before the patient was receiving the lactated Ringer's solution intravenously, with approximately 3,000 c.c. of the solution given daily. The only change, following the first intravenous feeding, was an addition of 20 milliequivalents of potassium chloride.

Throughout February 17 regular blood sugars were taken, an absolute necessity for a diabetic in such a condition. *By comparing her tremulous signs with the blood tests, it was definitely established that when her blood sugar was rising, the convulsions were less severe or even absent. When regular insulin was given, the convulsive seizures grew more severe.* Eventually this pattern moved toward a moment of even greater crisis: The blood sugar level was rising higher and higher, yet when insulin was given the patient would again go into convulsions. We were in a dilemma.

We had to keep her blood sugar level down to a safe standard. Insulin was the only means of doing so. But insulin seemed to be bringing on convulsions. One wondered if there was a way out.

At 4:00 P.M. that day—February 17—the patient went into convulsions that were so severe that two attendants had to hold her on the bed. Thirty minutes later her blood sugar was 260 milligrams percent, and her convulsions were so pronounced that I thought she would surely die. Something had to be done. At 5:50 P.M., hoping to depress her convulsive activity, I injected 20 c.c. of 10 percent magnesium sulfate into the vein, taking ten minutes to complete the injection. By the time the solution was completely injected, which was 6:00 P.M., she was sound asleep, her convulsions ended! At 6:07 P.M. there was a slight tremor of her legs, and then she went back to sleep.

At 6:15 P.M. the patient N. H. awoke and said, "Dr. Ellis, can I turn on my side?"

The nurse turned to me and said, "These are the first words she has spoken since I came on duty." The nurse had been in constant attendance for the past three hours and fifteen minutes.

Unassisted, and for the first time in several hours, the patient rearranged her bed covers, turned on her side, and went back to sleep.

This, to me, was sensational. Magnesium traditionally was classified as a depressant on the nervous system, and I had administered it for this reason, to halt the terrifying convulsions. What I had just witnessed, however, was not cerebral depression. It was *improved cerebration* brought about by magnesium therapy! Since the magnesium was the only change at all in her intravenous intake, it had to be given credit for the beneficial change that occurred.

Obviously, in this case pyridoxine had not been sufficient to halt or prevent convulsions, as it had done in other situations. Something different was at work in the diabetic patient. This was obvious in comparing N. H.'s ordeal with the relatively uncomplicated bowel-obstruction case of H. B. One must keep in mind that H. B. was older, had more adhesions, and went longer without food, yet she never convulsed. Quite clearly, insulin was directly associated with N. H.'s convulsions, and magnesium was intimately involved in stopping her signs and symptoms.

By this time N. H. had received, spread over the previous forty-eight hours, 6,000 c.c. of lactated Ringer's solution, by a continuous intravenous drip, that also included 300 milligrams of pyridoxine and other vitamins.

With the beneficial role of magnesium now evident to me, at 6:55 P.M. she was given 2 c.c. of 50 percent magnesium sulfate by intramuscular injection. At 7:00 P.M.—exactly one hour after the first injection of magnesium—the patient engaged in the most extended and significant conversation she had had in the past twenty-four hours.

She began flexing her fingers back and forth. "My fingers tingle and feel stiff," she said. "I'm trying to get the circulation back into them."

Very frankly, I thought the battle had been won.

Because her blood sugar at 7:00 P.M. was 276 milligrams percent—too high—she was given fifteen units of regular insulin fifteen minutes later, without ill effect. At 7:50 P.M. she was talking coherently with the nurse. Then, after arranging her bed covers, she went back to sleep.

During the ten-hour period lasting from 7:00 P.M. February 17 to 5:00 A.M. February 18, her nausea subsided and she did not vomit. She was fed a four-ounce solution of peanut butter in warm water through the Levin tube at four-hour intervals—at 8:00 P.M., midnight, and at 4:00 A.M. The tube was otherwise clamped throughout the night.

At 5:00 A.M. her blood sugar level was 216 milligrams percent, *and she was given ten units of regular insulin.* At 6:30 A.M., one and a half hours later, tremors began again in her legs. At 6:43 A.M. she was having violent convulsions that shook the entire bed. Again, 20 c.c. of 10 percent magnesium sulfate was given intravenously; at 7:05 A.M. she was again asleep.

All that day of February 18, each dose of insulin seemed to make the tremors worse, so that alternate injections of insulin and magnesium sulfate occurred. While the dilemma continued, the lactated Ringer's solution, with added vitamins and 20 milliequivalents of potassium chloride, proceeded as a slow intravenous drip.

The following excerpt (Fig. 8) from her hospital records shows the evaluation of her blood chemistries at noon on February 18.

That afternoon the patient became clearly conscious and talked normally. She still had received no relief from the pain in her abdomen, and the nausea and vomiting had continued. She begged to have something done about the intermittent cramping pain beneath the left subcostal margin, or under the lower rib region. There were audible bowel sounds that indicated a bowel obstruction.

Name **N.H.**				Date **2/18/72**		Rm. # **114**		Physician **Ellis**		
( ) Check test ordered in Square				□ Routine		□ CBC		□ Hgb-Hct	□ Wbc-Diff	
RBC	WBC		Hematocrit			Hgb		Gms		%
□ Retic		□ Platelets			□ Sed. Rate			mm/hrs.		

Schilling Differential	Count	Basos.	Eosins.	Myelos.	Juveniles	Stabs.	Segs.	Lymphs.	Monos	□ Serology
	Neutrophils, immature					mature				

□ Coag time		□ Bleeding time		□ Prothrombin		Sec. Control
□ Cell Indices — MCV			MCH		MCHC	
□ Blood type		Rh		□ Crossmatch	No. units	

CHEMISTRIES

Test	Normal	Result	Test	Normal	Result	Test	Normal	Result
□ Amylase	60-160		☑ Chlorides	99-108	**96**	☑ Potassium	4.1-5.6	**4.3**
□ BUN	8-18		□ Cholesterol (TOT)	140-250		☑ Sodium	135-152	**135**
□ Bilirubin (Dir)	0-0.2		☑ Glucose	80-120	**244**	□ SGO-T 1.	0-45	
Indirect	0.2-0.8		□ LDH	100-350		2.		
Total	0.2-1.2		□ Lipose	Up to 06		□ Total Protein	6.3-7.9	
□ BSP (45 min)	5% Ret.		□ Acid Phos.	0-0.9		□ Albumin	4.4-5.4	
☑ Calcium	4.5-5.5	**4.3**	□ Alk. Phos.	1.5-5.0		Globulin	1.8-3.2	
□ CO_2	20-30		□ Phosphorus	2.5-4.0		□ A/G Ratio		

LIST OTHER TEST DESIRED.

Technologist _____ *gov — 12 nddy 2/18/72*

Fig. 8.

With this background I took her into the operating room for surgery, and at 8:30 P.M. on February 18 I performed a laparotomy—opening the abdominal wall—and found the transverse colon obstructed by adhesions at the splenic flexure. Dissecting the adhesions free of the bowel, I closed the abdomen, hoping that the incessant vomiting and pain would be relieved, and it was.

The following day—February 19—despite the 1,000 milligrams of magnesium she was being given every eight hours by intramuscular injection, the patient began convulsing again.

Over and over again, as I had worried over the case for long, long hours, I puzzled over what was wrong. There seemed to be no pattern, no guidelines. The usual diabetic patient with either hyperglycemia or hypoglycemia did not convulse like this. It seemed that I had given enough magnesium, yet convulsions had recurred. Again, in desperation, she was given 20 c.c. of 10 percent magnesium sulfate intravenously. By this time the convulsions were shaking the bed. Following the injection, she slept a little while, then convulsions started up again.

At this point in her crisis a new thought occurred. I stopped the drip of lactated Ringer's solution.

In less than a minute the patient stopped convulsing!

Had the lactated Ringer's solution triggered the convulsions? If so, how did it do so? The questions were tantalizing. Except for preoperative medication and some narcotics for pain, all such medications were kept to an absolute minimum. A blood transfusion had been given following surgery, but the transfusion had been completed by the time the lactated Ringer's was resumed, accompanied by the recurrence of convulsions. The magnesium injections had been given to counteract the convulsions. Out of necessity the Levin tube had been left in the nose and into the stomach for several hours following the operation. This enabled the bowel to regain motility, thus avoiding abdominal distension. Sodium chloride, as normal saline, was then given intravenously, and the patient did not now convulse, even though insulin was also given.

Thirty-six hours after starting surgery, at 8:00 A.M. on February 20, N. H. was fed through the Levin tube three tablespoons of peanut butter dissolved in four ounces of water. The tube was then removed, and the patient was fed a soft, high-protein diet three times daily. The magnesium sulfate was continued, 1,000 milligrams by intramuscular injection at eight-hour intervals. The patient improved in strength and was free of vomiting.

At 1:00 P.M. on February 23 the patient felt well enough to sit on the side of her bed, and at 6:00 P.M. the same day she ate her meal and seemed to be improving. At 7:00 P.M. her blood sugar was 236 milligrams percent, there was a little acetone on her breath, and her skin was a bit dry. Accordingly I decided she needed some insulin and additional electrolytes. At 7:30 P.M. she was given 1,000 c.c. of lactated Ringer's solution by clysis (i.e., stuck in fat, not in the vein) with hyaluronidase, an enzyme that is squirted by tube to make it absorb faster. *This time the additional potassium chloride and vitamins were not included.*

At 7:55 P.M. she was given five units of insulin by hypodermic injection. At 2:00 A.M. on February 24 her right leg began shaking, and she began rolling her eyes back with a glaring stare. She rolled her head from side to side and for about sixty seconds she was stuporous. She vomited a small amount of mucus. Blood sugar at 3:45 A.M. was unchanged at 236 milligrams percent.

Again, it seemed that the lactated Ringer's had precipitated the convulsions. For more than three days and nights she had been improving—during which time she received no lactated Ringer's.

Following the last episode, she improved gradually, and she was discharged from the hospital on March 7. I subsequently saw her on April 2. She was in excellent spirits, feeling fine, with no complaints. She looked as if nothing had ever been wrong with her.

This case history has been given in such detail for two reasons: so that the biochemist reading it may further interpret the clinical significance of the findings, while non-doctors may gain some idea of the terrible nursing battle one has when a severely diabetic patient arrives in the emergency room with an acute bowel obstruction and an electrolyte imbalance.

The case of N. H. is revealing for what it teaches us on a number of points relating to the diabetic patient. Although hers is only one case, as is often true it tells us a great deal that can prove to be of value in the treatment of many other patients in the same medical predicament.

For four days and nights I virtually lived beside the patient's bedside. No effort was spared to save her life. At the same time I was making a sustained attempt to comprehend her convulsions, which looked exactly like those of eclampsia. As a result of this close vigil several observations became clear to me. On two points I was positive. First of all, when she received insulin, regardless of the glucose blood level, her convulsions were made worse. Secondly, the lactated Ringer's solution made the convulsions worse, and magnesium gave her remarkable relief from the convulsions.

I also arrived at several other opinions: When there is an electrolyte imbalance involving low blood magnesium, insulin precipitates convulsions. Furthermore, the primary effect of intravenous injection of concentrated magnesium sulfate, on a patient with eclampsia, is to change the magnesium-calcium ratio enough to halt production of insulin from the pancreas and thus halt the convulsive seizures. Additionally, B$_6$ deficiency contributes to brain hyperirritability, regardless of stimulus. From this data I was to conclude that unattended eclampsia is a convulsive state that results from two conditions operating simultaneously: hypomagnesemia (low blood magnesium) and vitamin B$_6$ deficiency.

N. H.'s forty-year-old son told me that he had never seen, or known of, his mother having convulsions except during these periods of stress in which a bowel obstruction was involved. The entire case, including his remark, sent me digging into the medical literature in an attempt to find the key to her problem. It seemed clear. Insulin triggered the convulsions, magnesium stopped them. Although I had earlier believed vitamin B$_6$ to be a particularly potent factor in relieving convulsions, especially as I had seen them in babies and in pregnant women, it appeared obvious that if B$_6$ had a role in N. H.'s recovery from convulsions, it was in conjunction with magnesium.

As I researched the literature I found at least a partial explanation for what I had seen happen to N. H. Two doctors, Warren E. C. Wacker and Alfred F. Parisi, in the *New England Journal of Medicine* in 1968, had reported: "Magnesium deficiency is relatively common in the postoperative period in association with prolonged nasogastric suction combined with administration of large amounts of magnesium-free parenteral fluids."[2]

Stripped of technical terminology, this was exactly what had happened to N. H. "Prolonged nasogastric suction"—that was the effect of the Levin tube that went through her nose on into her stomach. "Large amounts of magnesium-free parenteral fluids"— this was the lactated Ringer's solution that had electrolytes and vitamins but no magnesium. Without sufficient magnesium, N. H. had convulsed as if she had been a pregnant woman with eclampsia. Her convulsions were primarily tonic and clonic—that is, muscular contractions—in nature and never approached the *grand mal* seizure in intensity; nonetheless, they appeared to be the same type of convulsions that an obstetrician sees in a patient with eclampsia. It is, therefore, very likely that diabetic pregnant women, who are also in need of additional magnesium and who also must take insulin, also convulse because of the inadequate calcium-magnesium exchange at the cell level, a matter to be discussed in more detail in Chapter 11.

In the case of N. H., the magnesium was not a pharmacological (or extra large) dose, as seems to be commonly believed, but rather I believe it was replacing something that she had lost. This is particularly true for diabetic patients. In her own case, whatever level of magnesium she already had was further depleted by the nasogastric suction of the Levin tube. Wacker and Parisi have stated that such fluid contains about 1 milliequivalent per liter of magnesium. Removal of, let us say, 20 liters of fluid, plus the magnesium-free fluids such as in the Ringer's solution, could lead to quite low magnesium levels. This no doubt happened to this patient. The diabetic urinates frequently, and although the kidneys tend to conserve magnesium to a certain extent, this also contributes to a loss of magnesium, above that of other, non-diabetic patients.

Other clinical studies have statistically related low magnesium levels with diabetes. In one study Drs. Charles E. Jackson and Donald W. Meier determined by atomic absorption spectrophotometry, an exquisitely refined method for making quantitative measurements, the serum magnesium levels of 5,100 consecutive patients seen at their private general diagnostic clinic in Bluffton,

Indiana. A level of 1.53 to 1.99 milliequivalents per liter was chosen as the normal range, which included 90 percent of all patients examined. Of the diseases, diabetes mellitus was found to be the condition most frequently associated with hypomagnesemia, for 20 percent of patients with blood magnesium levels below 1.48 milliequivalents per liter had diabetes mellitus. The use of diuretics was also implicated by the study. Seven of eighteen patients—not necessarily diabetics—who had serum magnesium levels below 1.34 mEq/L had been taking diuretics of some kind.[3] Wacker and Parisi have also reviewed the damage that diuretics may do by depleting the patient's magnesium in his body.

A few years ago the old concept that magnesium is a central-nervous-system depressant was challenged by G. Somjen, M. Hilmy, and C. R. Stephen in work at Dallas's Parkland Memorial Hospital. Two of the researchers took enough magnesium sulfate to raise the serum level to 15 milliequivalents per liter, approximately ten times that of the control values. It caused temporary neuromuscular paralysis. However, the patients did not lose consciousness, and they did not lose their perception to pain.[4] Based on my observation of N. H., as well as this experiment by Somjen and colleagues, it is my opinion that magnesium is associated with the sleep mechanism and that correction of hypomagnesemia, in association with adequate vitamin B₆, improves sleep. This was apparent in N. H.'s case, for it not only produced increased cerebration in her case, but it also stopped her convulsions and enabled her to rest, including going into a restful sleep.

At the cellular level, potassium, calcium, and magnesium are involved in constant exchanges. Calcium and sodium are outside the cell; magnesium, inside the cell. Insulin is the driving force that moves these electrolytes about, and magnesium, in particular, is intimately associated with carbohydrate metabolism in the brain. My diabetic patient N. H. surely was in need of magnesium. When calcium was given in the lactated Ringer's solution that had 200 milligrams of calcium chloride per liter and no magnesium, convulsions occurred. In retrospect this seems obvious. In a review of magnesium metabolism, Wacker and Parisi have reported tetany, or muscular spasms, in animals with low magnesium levels in their blood. Babies have convulsed after losing magnesium as a result of prolonged diarrhea followed by a cow's-milk diet; the milk, containing much calcium but little magnesium, caused further depletion of magnesium because the calcium crowded out the magnesium in the race for absorption. (The competitiveness of the two ions will be discussed in Chapter 11.) They also noted that, with the diabetic during insulin and fluid therapy, the serum magnesium concentration falls rapidly. On the other hand one study of one hundred patients with controlled diabetes revealed that serum magnesium rose significantly with age from normal levels to a mean high of 2.33 milliequivalents per liter in those over sixty years of age. Why this happened is not clear. But what is clear is that, generally, diabetics and those persons receiving diuretics are likely to have lower blood levels of magnesium—sufficiently low, in some patients, to trigger convulsions.

But how, one may ask, does this involve vitamin B_6, about which this book is written? B_6 and magnesium are intimately related. In clinical observations it may not be clear that the 300 milligrams of pyridoxine N. H. was getting were interacting with the injections of magnesium, even though it may be shown in a laboratory. Yet magnesium and B_6 are co-factors. How do they work together? For the non-doctor it may be expressed in this manner: Some of these chemical bindings that take place in the body are very flimsy and loose. If one could visualize two bales of cotton floating in space, held together with a cockleburr, then B_6 might be pictured in some of these magnesium reactions as the cockleburr. The attachment is there, but is ever so delicate.

What is of paramount importance is that magnesium determination is not a part of the routine blood chemistries taken in hospitals today. Yet the serum magnesium is as important as any other mineral that may be evaluated, and in the diabetic patient it is absolutely necessary that the lab test for magnesium levels.

As for B_6 therapy for diabetes mellitus, it is yet to be proved conclusively that pyridoxine benefits all patients suffering from diabetes. I cannot state that B_6 reduces the amount of insulin a diabetic may require. I tried to prove this but did not. At the same time, most diabetics, as I have seen in my own practice, do find relief from signs and symptoms accompanying diabetes, such as neuritis and neuropathies and edema, and because of this, B_6 supplementation, along with additional magnesium, is recommended for the diabetic with the knowledge that it cannot worsen his condition and may very possibly help him. And based on Kotake's experiments with laboratory animals there is also a good chance that an adequate supply of B_6 will help prevent diabetes.

Heart Disease and B₆ | 10

Early in the nineteen sixties I was called to the bedside of G. R.,
a fifty-two-year-old woman I had known for many years. As a
young woman she and her husband had lived on my father's ranch,
where her husband had once been the foreman. The husband was
concerned that afternoon because his wife was nauseated—"sick
at her stomach."

As I sat beside her bed and talked with her I was struck by
an observation that she didn't complain of, didn't even mention.
Her cheeks were almost glistening. They were puffed, not around
her eyes but in her cheeks, and her hands were also puffed.

I examined her chest and abdomen, but I remained puzzled over
the nausea. Any of a half dozen conditions could have caused it.
I wrote a prescription for some tablets that would relieve the
symptoms of nausea and then I asked her, "How long have your
hands and face been puffed?"

She didn't know they were puffed.

I looked more intently at her face. *In the front of the cheek-
bones, where the elastic connective tissues make the cheeks
prominent, the skin seemed to be most puffed and most shiny.*

"Did you ever notice anything unusual about your hands?" I
asked her.

"At times, for two or three nights in a row," she said, "I would feel like I was asleep all over. My arms and hands would feel numb, and I could get the fingers moving and the blood seemed to circulate, and the numbness would go away."

"Do you ever have any pains in your legs?"

"Yes."

"When?"

"I have to get out of bed at night and rub the cramps from the backs of my legs." And then she mentioned a symptom that fascinated me: "I have had that tingling in the right cheek of my face and along my jaw and up toward my ear. The first time I noticed it, I was pregnant with my first baby. I had that tingling in the cheek of my face both times I was pregnant."

"What do you eat ordinarily during the week?" I asked her.

"I've used cooking oil to fry foods for three or four years," she said, naming a very popular brand name of a polyunsaturated fat cooking oil. "I did all of my frying with cooking oil, except my eggs. I would use bacon grease left in the skillet for frying eggs. For several years we've used margarine instead of cow butter. I never drank sweet milk except when I ate cereals. We had beefsteak every day, pork chops once a week, and chicken once a week. I always ate the fat off the meat because I like it. My husband and boys ate the lean meat, and I ate the fat." She and her husband had eaten from the same table for four decades.

On my way back to town that day I realized she had described the usual paresthesia of B₆ deficiency and had mentioned the severe leg cramps that also afflict the B₆-deficient person. She was the first patient, among a number who were discovered later, who noticed a tingling that radiated along her jaw and into the cheek of her face. Her condition had been accentuated by her two pregnancies. What was most important to me was that she mentioned this paresthesia along her jaw. It had been accepted that paresthesia along the jaw may be associated with angina pectoris. Was it possible that the associated paresthesia might be heralding an oncoming catastrophe? If this could be shown to be true, then through use of B₆ we could take a giant step toward prevention of heart disease, which was then killing Americans by the hundreds of thousands each year.

G. R., at fifty-two, was, in other words, past the age of meno-pause. She had had the same tingling in her cheek during her two pregnancies.[1]

It was no accident that I thought of angina pectoris in connection with G. R.'s case, for with angina pectoris there is often paresthesia of the hands and particularly of the little fingers. As William Heberden had published (posthumously) in London in 1802, "There is numbness and swelling in the arm." "Angina pectoris" was a syndrome of chest pain associated with acute anxiety, which Heberden first described and named. (Heberden in 1767 had become the first to distinguish between chicken pox and smallpox.)

"Some," wrote Heberden, "have been seized while they were standing still, or sitting, also upon first waking out of sleep; and the pain sometimes reaches to the right arm, as well as to the left, and even down to the hands, but this is uncommon; in a very few instances the arm has at the same time been numbed and swelled. In one or two persons the pain has lasted some hours, or even days; but this has happened when the complaint has been of long standing, and thoroughly rooted in the constitution. . . . The termination of angina pectoris is remarkable. For if no accident intervene, but the disease go to its height, the patients all suddenly fall down, and perish almost immediately. Of which indeed their frequent faintness, and sensations as if all the powers of life were failing, afford no obscure intimation."[2]

Although Heberden's primary interest was in the chest pain that often presaged the violent myocardial infarction of which his patients died, he came very close to a description of other symptoms—arm pain, numbness in the hands, and swelling in the hands—that I was to find responsive to B$_6$. A large number of my patients since G. R. have had this swelling and numbness with angina pectoris, and these symptoms responded to B$_6$ therapy. The pain in some instances was relieved; in others it definitely was not. But they were improved enough to indicate that B$_6$ should be taken by patients suffering from angina pectoris.

(A grim postscript to the G. R. case is that seven years later her husband died of acute myocardial infarction at the age of sixty-four.)

From as early as November 1961 as I was at the beginning of my clinical studies, there was one symptom that kept recurring in the data I collected from patients: vague chest pain. Usually the chest pain was one that radiated from the chest into the arm or from the arm into the chest. As it involved the arm it reminded me of angina pectoris, which leads one on to the whole subject of heart attacks.

Most persons think of a "heart attack" as a very dangerous, often acute and fatal episode of heart disease, characterized by crushing chest pain, profuse sweating, extreme paleness, profound prostration, and shock. At one time this condition was called "acute indigestion," because nausea and vomiting also accompany it. Later it was called "coronary artery thrombosis," denoting that a blood clot had hit the main artery that feeds the heart muscle. About the same time a term, "coronary occlusion," was developed; this meant the artery was blocked inside by a clot or by deposits of calcium and cholesterol. In more recent years a new term, "myocardial infarction," has come into use, indicating heart muscle has died. A myocardial infarction is an acute heart attack in which there is a sudden ischemic dying of heart muscle for no known reason. Infarction refers to the dead area that suddenly occurs. As yet it has not been explained. "Myocardial infarction" is preferred by the cardiologists because it is now known that heart muscle can suddenly die without arteriosclerosis, although this is very rare, and without a proved occlusion. Why? That is still the puzzle before us.

There are many mysteries in the study of heart disease. One cannot say that every person with angina pectoris will eventually suffer, or die from, a myocardial infarction or a coronary artery thrombosis, but it is reasonable to assume that where there is smoke there is also fire. As a rule, angina pectoris precedes myocardial infarction by a number of years.

There are several facts that perplex doctors. There is autopsy evidence to support the view that myocardial infarction is not always associated with arteriosclerosis. Nor is the electrocardiogram (EKG) an infallible detector of myocardial infarction. For example, a patient may have an EKG that is typical of one associated with myocardial infarction—and he may not have myocardial infarction. At the same time, it is possible for a person to suffer myocardial infarction and die without having had any chest pain. Obviously, doctors found it difficult to fit these aberrant pieces into the heart-disease picture.

In many instances, however, myocardial infarction was preceded by arm and chest pains of varying intensity and duration, and it was this chest pain in my fat-eating patients that first drew me into this sphere of clinical research. It was a complicated, serendipitous path: In seeking the cause of "the heart attack," I had instituted dietary changes in my patients. This had led to studying other, seemingly unrelated signs and symptoms ranging from rheumatism to the edema of pregnancy. But through some of the associated symptoms that responded to B_6 therapy, a suspicious trail led back to heart disease. And so, beginning with an interest in fat metabolism and cholesterol my studies led to a single vitamin, thence back to some early observed symptoms.

Now, after eleven years of investigations that have ranged far afield in the human body, it is quite clear that a number of these signs and symptoms that respond to B_6 are also part of the burden of the heart patient. Patients with heart disease almost invariably have problems with fluid retention and excretion. This is edema. To some degree this can be treated by B_6. It is granted that this edema and the edema, say, of pregnancy may be of unrelated etiology or cause, but edema is edema, and that which can be relieved with a vitamin—whether it be the edema of scurvy, beriberi, pellagra, or an increased need for B_6—should be relieved by the appropriate vitamin.

Of utmost importance is the fact that "coronary prone" individuals have many of the signs and symptoms that I have been describing in this book. Edema, numbness and tingling, disturbance of hand grip, and inability to perform the QEW test—patients with these are "coronary prone." From studying these patterns over the past decade I have been able to anticipate myocardial infarction in a number of patients, several of whom are now dead from that very disorder. Several of the patients whose detailed cases I gave in my earlier book, *The Doctor Who Looked at Hands,* died of cardiovascular disease within five years of the book's publication.

Here at the outset it must be stated emphatically that pyridoxine will not prevent myocardial infarction in the strictest sense of analysis. If a disease has been building up for decades, a few years of therapy can't be expected to counteract and wipe out all the long years of damage. I have treated patients who had been taking pyridoxine daily for months or even years and they dropped dead of myocardial infarction. One can reasonably conclude that some disease conditions, such as, for instance, arteriosclerosis, eventually reach an irreversible stage. In these cases the best that can be done, often, is to prevent further deterioration, and this is not so easily done.

What, then, is the clinical association between B$_6$ deficiency and a heart attack of the myocardial infarction type? Three short case histories will suggest some insight.

J. S., sixty-two, was a carpenter whose right hand became numb, weakened, swollen, and painful as he was driving nails with a hammer while working on a barn. During the week of July 6, 1964, he was observed by three physicians, including an orthopedist, and a diagnosis of "carpal tunnel syndrome" was made. One recommended that the hand be operated on, resecting the transverse carpal ligament. This was before my later conclusions about carpal tunnel syndrome. I observed that he had swelling in the right hand and that his QEW test was also positive for his left hand. He had thick, puffy hands. On the basis of this, on July 10 I prescribed 50 milligrams of pyridoxine a day, and he continued work as well as he could.

"After three weeks," J. S. said, "the feeling came back in my hand. It was sixty to ninety days before feeling was completely normal."

All edema had subsided in both hands. He had regained full flexion of his fingers in both hands. Relieved by pyridoxine of the symptoms related to his thick, puffy, edematous hands, he continued to build houses and barns for more than seven years, obviously a very active carpenter, until November 3, 1971, when he suffered a massive myocardial infarction.

Following admission to the hospital, he developed ventricular fibrillation, a cardiac arrhythmia. It is characterized by an absolutely irregular spread of idiocentricular excitation whose origin and spread are completely disordered. It produces only limited, ineffectual, and irregular ventricular contractions. Being almost always irreversible, it usually is fatal.

His heart quit beating. While a nurse and a medical colleague administered closed cardiac massage, I performed a tracheotomy to provide mechanical artificial respiration. ("First time I ever cut a man's throat with him looking at me," I kidded him afterward in the hospital when he was out of danger.) Fortunately, he survived, and he was discharged from the hospital on December 10.

During these seven years J. S. had been taking 50 milligrams of pyridoxine daily. It had not, then, prevented a heart attack that had almost taken his life. But what is of deep interest to us is that following his heart attack, and for the next several months, he sustained a loss of sensation, or hypoesthesia, in the left hand stretching from the crease of the wrist to the tips of the ring and little fingers. This is the exact distribution of the ulnar nerve. The symptom, coming directly in association with the heart attack, definitely links his myocardial infarction to the nervous system and leads me to conclude that, whatever the role of the circulatory system in heart disease, the nervous system is intimately involved. Whatever had damaged his heart muscle had very likely in some way also affected his ulnar nerve. *I was almost positive that there had been a tightening of ligaments in the hand through which the ulnar nerve passed.*

During that same month, November 1971, in another room of the same hospital, another patient, F. H., lay flat on his back in an oxygen tent. F. H., fifty-nine, a husky cattleman, had also suffered a myocardial infarction.

He also had had a history of numbness, tingling, and swelling in his hands and fingers, which he had reported in April 1967—four years before. In 1967 his hands were thick and "puffy" in appearance. His positive QEW test showed maximum flexion of his fingers to be not more than 50 percent. The numbness and tingling in his hands had persisted during both day and night. During the next six weeks on pyridoxine (50 milligrams daily), both he and

I were struck by a truly remarkable reduction of edema in his hands; the numbness and tingling subsided, and his finger flexion returned to normal.

Two years later, in 1969, F. H. began having paroxysmal tachycardia, or "fast heart," and he was given quinidine, and his pyridoxine dosage was increased to 100 milligrams daily.

But in November 1971 he went to the hospital with acute myocardial infarction. Fortunately he survived and was discharged from the hospital.

A third case is that of B. S., seventy-one, a retired cattleman who on May 1, 1969, complained of "chest pain." His pain had become progressively worse for the past five years. Along with his chest pains he had had a gradually progressive stiffness of his arms, shoulders, and hands. His fingers in recent months had become very painful to pressure, and a handshake brought excruciating pain to his fingers. He said he had lost sensation in his fingers to the degree that he couldn't, by perception when his eyes were closed, distinguish cloth, wood, or glass.

X-ray pictures revealed calcifications of the abdominal aorta and arthritis of the lumbar vertebrae. He had an irregular heart rhythm, with a rate of ninety-six beats per minute. At the suggestion of another physician he had been taking three grains of quinidine twice daily. His urine was negative for sugar and albumin.

Edema was manifest in this man. His feet and legs had a pitting edema above the ankles, and there was a glistening white sheen of tight shiny skin over his finger joints, and diffuse swelling of both hands. As a part of the gross deformity of both hands, he had an advanced stiffness and loss of function in all fingers at the interphalangeal joints. Moving his arms caused him great pain at the shoulders.

In short, B. S. had chest pain, calcification of his arteries, arthritis of his vertebral joints, the "shoulder-hand" syndrome, cardiac decompensation with a rapid rate, edema of the feet and ankles, and moist rales in his lungs. He was what I had grown accustomed to thinking of as a "coronary-prone" patient with existing *cardiac decompensation*. He also had signs and symptoms that I knew, on the basis of experience with thousands of other patients, would respond to pyridoxine. I instructed him to discontinue the quinidine and to take 50 milligrams of pyridoxine night and morning.

Six weeks later, on June 15, 1969, he had a remarkable reduction of pain in his hands and fingers. Some deformity was still present, however, and it was to remain as a result of what seemed to be irreversible arthritic changes in the interphalangeal joints. (Even three years later he couldn't make a fist.) Without a doubt, swelling was completely eliminated in both hands, and it did not recur. The sensation in his fingertips had returned to normal so that he could close his eyes and distinguish between glass, wood, and cloth by touch only. In his feet and ankles, edema was still present, but it was considerably less than when he had first entered the office, back in early May.

At this time he was told how to take digitalis, and digitalization was begun. By his next visit on August 11 he had no edema in the feet and legs and no moist rales in his lungs. Ten and a half months after beginning treatment with pyridoxine, on March 15, 1970, he was taking one and a half grains of digitalis and 50 milligrams of pyridoxine daily. His fingers and hands were free of pain and paresthesia. The tactile sensation in his fingers was normal. He was devoid of edema in his feet and ankles and of rales in his lungs. He had some residual pain in the shoulders, but less than at the beginning. His fingers had shown slow but gradual improvement in flexibility. His heart rate was eighty beats per minute.

My diagnosis was that this old cattleman, B. S., had rheumatism, the shoulder-hand syndrome, and to some degree edema that were all responsive to pyridoxine. In addition, he had congestive heart failure with additional edema that required digitalization. In short, he had one type of edema that was responsive to B₆, and he had another edema that was responsive to digitalis. I have observed this combination of edema in numbers of elderly cardiac patients.

Returning to the cases of J. S. and F. H., the two men who had received pyridoxine for years and who were in the hospital at the same time with myocardial infarction, one might suggest that if vitamin B₆ deficiency contributed to their narrow brush with death, then it had played its role much earlier in life, or even before they were born, during those extremely important nine months of fetal life. Each one had a family history reflecting heart disease. The cattleman F. H. had a sister who dropped dead while ironing clothes, and she too had been taking pyridoxine. The carpenter J. S. had a brother who died of myocardial infarction. I had also treated the carpenter J. S.'s brother. The brother experienced the same truly spectacular reduction of edema in his hands when he, too, was given pyridoxine before digitalis. Several months later the man died of myocardial infarction. Was I locking the barn after the horse was gone? In advanced cases such as these, one tends to think so.

The case of the first patient, J. S., suggests that when there is a long-standing need for vitamin B₆ one can expect progressive changes in all ligaments and bands of connective tissues in the hand. It will be recalled that he earlier had had a diagnosis of carpal tunnel syndrome in his right hand, which was relieved by B₆; later, at the time of his heart attack, he suffered hypoesthesia of that part of his left hand that was supplied by the ulnar nerve. As seen in Chapter 4, the branches of the ulnar nerve to the ring and little finger do not pass through the carpal tunnel, but the tendon sheath or synovia of the little finger does pass under the transverse carpal ligament. This is indication enough that paresthesia in the hand is not only associated with swelling of synovia but is also secondary to constriction of ligaments in the palm. It is my opinion that much of the vague chest pain and pain around the shoulders and upper arms in these patients with rheumatism and heart disease is the result of constriction of nerves by ligaments and other dense connective tissues. Also, the sympathetic nerves in the neck and chest, anatomically speaking, are literally surrounded by dense bands of connective tissue.

The electrocardiograms (EKGs) (Figs. 9 and 10) are those of J. S. and F. H., shown as a matter of interest to document the fact of their heart attacks. Although the squiggles and tracings may be esoteric to non-doctors, any doctor will understand that the T-waves in these EKGs indicate these men had myocardial infarctions.

The seventy-five-bed general hospital where these patients were treated, the Titus County Memorial Hospital, Mt. Pleasant, Texas, is staffed by nine physicians. For several years all electrocardio-

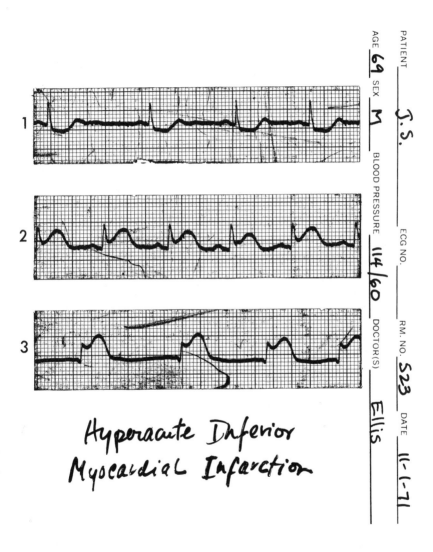

Fig. 9. Electrocardiogram of patient J. S.

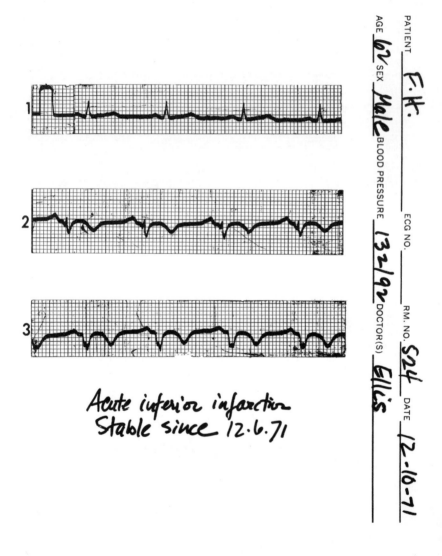

Fig. 10. Electrocardiogram of patient F. H.

grams made there had been interpreted by Dr. Vanis Pennington, an internal-medicine specialist trained at the Henry Ford Hospital in Detroit, Michigan. In 1970, after observing my and others' patients for three years, Dr. Pennington stated for the record: "Patients who had myocardial infarctions and who received pyridoxine had less deviation of the S-T segment in their electrocardiograms."

As a further difference in patients who had been taking pyridoxine, Dr. Pennington often found it difficult to determine if my patients had myocardial infarction or angina pectoris, because changes in the S-T segment of their EKGs were more fleeting. In order to verify the diagnosis of myocardial infarction by data to support the EKG, he had also to depend on transaminase elevation, temperature elevation, white blood count elevation, and general appearance of the patient. Transaminase is the enzyme that catalyzes the transfer of the amino group of a dicarboxylic amino acid to a keto acid, to form another amino acid.

For the last five years, as a matter of routine I have given 100 milligrams of pyridoxine by injection and 40 milliequivalents of potassium by mouth to numbers of patients arriving in the emergency room with acute myocardial infarction. I asked Dr. Pennington whether, in his opinion, it was the potassium or the pyridoxine that had decreased deviations of the S-T segment in my patients' EKGs. He replied that he often gave his own patients potassium, but he didn't see the same degree of improvement in their EKGs that he had seen in those who also took pyridoxine. Although it is a matter that is difficult to prove to anyone's satisfaction, I believe this routine treatment has reduced the mortality rate of my patients. This demonstrated difference in the electrocardiograms is sufficient to conclude that pyridoxine improves electrical conduction in the heart that has suffered a recent infarction. This seems to be sufficient justification for using B$_6$ in treating patients who have suffered myocardial infarctions.

As I have already stated in this chapter—but perhaps it needs reiterating—one cannot say that persons taking pyridoxine do not have myocardial infarctions. I have had patients die with myocardial infarction who had been receiving daily doses of B$_6$. But, invariably, they were patients who had advanced arteriosclerosis or diabetes and who also exhibited the symptomatology that I have described, such as paresthesia of the hands, edema of the hands, nocturnal muscle spasms, and impaired finger flexion. This, of course, is a major reason for designating the finger-flexion exercise as the Quick Early Warning test, for it may well prove to be one of the first clues in singling out the coronary-prone patient.

Several points are pertinent when discussing the heart attack itself. The same electrolytes mentioned in previous chapters—magnesium, potassium, sodium, and very likely calcium—must be in a state of equilibrium for the heart to function properly. This is true not only in the heart muscle but also in the nerves that go to the heart muscle. There is an acid-alkali relationship that is also important in this electrolyte exchange.

It should also be taken into account that women do not have myocardial infarctions until after menopause, whereas after menopause they begin to have heart attacks at the same ratio as men. Here again, as I pointed out in the chapters on pregnancy, menopause and menstruation, and the birth-control pill, is the female hormone relationship—a relationship in which B_6 very likely plays a vital role. Certainly, as has been shown over and over, B_6 does play a vital role in the estrogen-related disorders already examined. It seems possible the same may be true, at least to some extent, of the heart attack.

What is frequently overlooked, and is rarely known by non-doctors, is that in the urine of men there is half as much estrone, so-called female hormone, as there is in the urine of women. Estrone is the excreted form of estrogen. Where does this female hormone, estrogen, come from in the male? It comes from the male testicle. An authority on endocrinology, Dr. Arthur Grollman, in discussing the presence of estrogen in the testis, has written: "The average daily urinary excretion of estrogen corresponds to from 9 to 12 micrograms of estrone in men and from 18 to 36 in women. The estrogenic substance in male urine resembles estrone in certain respects. The significance of estrogens in the male organism is still unknown."[3]

This provides us with another possible loose association between estrogen imbalance with other hormones and a need for B_6 in metabolism. Investigators for years have been searching for a relationship of hormone imbalance and coronary thrombosis because there was no doubt that women are ordinarily spared the affliction of coronary thrombosis—and myocardial infarction, to use the now commonly preferred term—until after the menopause. It seemed possible, in my experience, that the neuritis-arthritis condition, seen in the patient who had had a heart attack, was the same arthritis-neuritis that often accompanied menopause, as well as disorders related to menstruation and the antiovulatory pills. If this were so, it left the great possibility that both conditions would respond to B_6.

As everyone knows, there are other major, accepted considerations in heart disease. Arteriosclerosis is the obviously big one. It is true that a person may not have arteriosclerosis, or he may not have very much arteriosclerosis, and he may still have a myocardial infarction. But this is not the pattern. It must be recognized that arteriosclerosis is the prime factor in the deadly myocardial infarction—and researchers in at least two laboratories have demonstrated, independently of each other, that *arteriosclerosis was caused in experimental animals by diets that were deficient in vitamin B_6.*

Drs. James F. Rinehart and Louis D. Greenberg, of the University of California School of Medicine in San Francisco in 1949, more than twenty years ago, described arteriosclerotic lesions in B_6-deficient monkeys. In 1952, reporting in *Circulation*, Rinehart and Henry D. Moon, another pathologist at the University of California, found that hardening of the arteries starts with deposits of mucuslike material in the lining of the blood-vessel walls. This reversed the beliefs that the fatty steroid, cholesterol, was first deposited. In the findings of Rinehart and Moon, cholesterol and other fatty chemicals are laid down later in the mucoid formations. They also found that the mucoid deposits are progressive with age but not necessarily a normal process. These findings indicated that arteriosclerosis is more related to the metabolism of protein than to fat, as had been widely believed. These pathological findings closely paralleled the experimental results that Rinehart and Greenberg had got in their feeding tests with monkeys on B_6-deficient diets, which produced arterioscleroticlike lesions. Rinehart and Moon based their 1952 report on studies of the arteries of 250 persons, some of whom had died of coronary thrombosis.

In other experiments, Gladys A. Emerson of the School of Public Health, University of California at Los Angeles, had virtually the same results with experimental dogs on B_6-deficient diets. Scientists, in all, have proved that monkeys, dogs, and chickens on B_6-deficient diets develop arterial changes that are in keeping with those of arteriosclerosis in the human being. Control animals did not develop the lesions. In the nineteen sixties, accelerated arteriosclerosis was found in *children,* in association with an inborn metabolic error.

The results from the laboratory, to be discussed in more detail in Chapter 11, definitely point toward vitamin B_6 deficiency as a prime factor in development of coronary arteriosclerosis. In the clinic, including my own work, it has not been proved that the heart attack can be prevented by pyridoxine. But it has been proved, certainly in my own clinic, that numbers of patients who had objective response to vitamin B_6 were coronary-prone individuals who subsequently suffered myocardial infarction. It goes without saying that it is much more difficult to prove that many, many coronary-prone patients were given pyridoxine in time to head off deadly myocardial infarctions.

For many years clinicians have been aware that a form of arthritis appears and becomes more pronounced either at the time of acute myocardial infarction or during the period of convalescence following the heart attack. We have seen this association in cases already presented in this chapter. This form of arthritis, which can more properly be described as the "shoulder-hand syndrome," is characterized primarily by edema of the hands and fingers, stiffness, pain and impaired flexion of the hands and fingers, and painful movement of the elbows and shoulders. In the past, treatment for this consisted of analgesics and steroids to provide symptomatic relief of pain. But now it has been demonstrated that B_6 will provide varying degrees of relief, indicating the strong possibility that B_6 deficiency in the first instance was the cause of the syndrome.

On the basis of observations I have already recorded in this book it would appear that vitamin B_6 is preventive and therapeutically specific for the "shoulder-hand syndrome." As I studied the pattern expressed by the cases of many patients I was able to see a sequence of symptoms and signs that developed insidiously over a long period of time before the shoulder-hand syndrome was fully manifest. At first the fingers became incompletely flexed, and there was edema in the hands before the patients themselves were aware of their hands becoming incapacitated. On the heels of paresthesia came motor-power failure and weakness of hand grip, and later there were disturbed tactile sensations in the fingers.

In a number of cases there was some weakness of hand grip long before pain developed in their shoulders and elbows. Sooner or later the patient noticed stiffness and pain in his shoulders and elbows, often suddenly after exercise; it was then, when the symptoms finally became severe, that he sought medical attention.

The age of the patient and the length of time he had been incapacitated had a great deal of effect on his response to therapy, but *some* sign or symptom improved in *every* patient treated with pyridoxine for the shoulder-hand syndrome. This is important. Since clinicians have, for a long time, considered the shoulder-hand syndrome to be a sequela, or a resultant disease condition, of the acute heart attack of the myocardial infarction type, B$_6$ becomes important in treatment of patients recovering from acute myocardial infarction.

In speaking of the cases in this book I have frequently used the word "stiffness" in describing symptoms. Now I wish to draw attention to the opposite of that term—that is to say, "spring, stretch, and recoil." I have already described the arterial changes in laboratory animals that compare with those of arteriosclerosis, or hardening of the arteries, in the human being. Just as much as the fingers have stiffness, so do the arteries in arteriosclerosis exhibit stiffness. An artery must have elasticity for pulsation and function, and nerves and tendons also depend on elasticity for movement at the joints. It is hoped that biochemists and animal physiologists will continue the exploration of enzymatic reactions that have to do with this elasticity of tissues, and elastic connective tissue in particular. It appears that there is swelling, not necessarily edema, in the elastic connective tissues of the cheeks of the face in association with B$_6$ deficiency.

For years now medical science, in researching for causes of heart disease, has concentrated on the circulatory system and the fatty deposits in the arterial walls. In this way cholesterol, for instance, has been linked to arteriosclerosis and heart disease. However, it might be well to shift the emphasis in another direction now. There are no doubts that deposits are plugging up the arteries of persons suffering from heart disease. But there is more to it than that.

During my medical career I have performed more than eight hundred autopsies, and one thing I have noted about healthy tissue is its elasticity. In an autopsy, one can cut a nerve or a blood vessel in two and tug at it with the fingers. Healthy nerves or blood vessels will snap back, like rubber bands. They are elastic. But in cases of arteriosclerosis this does not happen. In St. Louis, during my residency in surgery and pathology while I was doing autopsies, I found that almost everybody over fifty years of age had a yellow, gritty, rocklike substance in the walls of their heart arteries. Many arteries were actually as hard as rocks and felt like tubular rocks. They couldn't function because the elastic fibers and muscle fibers that give a young blood vessel snap and spring were gone. Under the microscope one could see that the slender elastic fibers, which ordinarily look like slivers of rubber, were replaced by calcium deposits. That condition is called hardening of the arteries. These blood vessels had lost their snap, indicating that the pathology of these cases is concerned primarily with the walls and the tissues of the blood vessels themselves rather than with what is deposited inside them.

Although this has never been suggested before, to my knowledge, I believe that the key to heart disease is to be found in the elastic fibers of the blood vessels. It further seems logical that adequate intake of B₆ throughout life would help insure continued elasticity of these vessels, just as B₆ does the same for other fibers, such as in the hands, that are involved in the processes of "spring, stretch, and recoil."

It is a far leap from rheumatism or arthritic condition in the hands to myocardial infarction, but it is important to recognize that these clinical observations did not come in a jump but in gradual, small steps, as any such conclusion must be made. Eventually, a direct association was established.

As I have indicated earlier, my investigations into this area began, logically enough, with observing the arthritic conditions that followed the heart attack. By then I had already proved that B₆ relieved the signs and symptoms in other patients who had not had heart attacks. It seemed sensible to take the same approach for the same signs and symptoms in the patients who had had heart attacks. Until that time, so far as I know, there had been no specific treatment for this arthritic condition.

My first investigation was of ten patients who had arthritis of the hands and who had histories of having had recent myocardial infarction. I sought to determine if B₆, as pyridoxine hydrochloride, would relieve this arthritis of the hands and fingers, based on treatment with 50 to 100 milligrams of pyridoxine daily. Effects would be measured by before-and-after observations.

The results were very encouraging. Within two weeks edema of the hands was relieved in all ten patients. Tendons were again conspicuous on the backs of their hands. Edema of the feet and ankles also subsided. By the end of three weeks there was a reduction in their wincing during an ordinary handshake. In most cases the patients could flex their fingertips to the metacarpophalangeal creases of the palms, with the QEW test. This provided objective proof of B₆-relieved arthritic symptoms and signs that were related to post-myocardial infarction. It also seemed certain that they were simultaneously suffering from either vitamin B₆ deficiency or had an increased need for B₆.

One of my earliest insights into a new approach to the heart attack came with the fatal illness of one of my patients in the early sixties. W. S., a long-time patient of mine, had come to the hospital one day in agony because of impaired circulation in his left leg and foot. The foot was white and cold, with no pulsation in the artery on top of his foot. The options facing me, to relieve his agony, were clear but not easy: either amputation of the leg or a lumbar sympathectomy, hoping to relieve his pain. I chose the complicated operation on the lumbar sympathetic nerve, hoping to save his leg. The ganglia of the sympathetic and parasympathetic nerves were dissected and removed from their location adjacent to the back vertebra on the left side. It was a success. Before W. S. left the operating table his left foot was as warm and as pink as a baby's foot. For the next ten months he had use of his leg, long enough to raise a corn crop. In fact, he paid his doctor's bill with seventy-five bushels of that corn.

But the operation, it appeared, only postponed the unpleasant inevitable. Arteriosclerosis of leg arteries continued, and the condition in his legs deteriorated eventually. In time, nothing short of amputation could help him, and both legs were amputated. W. S. became a double amputee because of arteriosclerosis.

Some time after that W. S. reported a new symptom. His little finger hurt him when he "bumped" the bed covers, so sensitive was it. This was before I had realized B_6 was the vitamin in the Morrison diet that was helping my patients specifically, and I had placed him on the low-cholesterol diet. His symptoms were relieved by the diet. Now the little finger's sensitivity suggested the ulnar nerve was involved, as it has been seen to be in cases of other patients since W. S.

In early 1962 W. S. hobbled down to his barn on his artificial legs. He became nauseated. When he got back to the house he sat down in the kitchen. His face turned white and he broke out into what his wife described as "a cold sweat." Then he developed pain in his chest, and his wife called me. I hurried out to the farm, but he died before I could see him.

He had had arteriosclerosis in his legs, and he must surely have died of arteriosclerosis in his heart arteries.

It is commonly known by doctors that when a blood vessel on the back side of the heart is blocked by thrombosis or a clot the patient is more likely to have tingling hands than when the clot occurs on the front side of the heart. Also, a clot on the back side of the heart is more dangerous, because it damages more heart nerves. In the early years of my investigations, out of the hundreds of patients I saw with tingling hands, three stood out as not completely relieved by B_6. All three had suffered severe thromboses of the coronary arteries. Those three men had lowered blood pressures as the result of their heart muscles having been weakened. Although they all regained enough strength to recover and return to work, they continued to have tingling sensations, first in one hand and then in the other, when they would sit down with their elbows resting on the arms of a chair and elevate their hands to the level of their faces.

After eleven years of correlating B_6 deficiency with acute myocardial infarction, I acknowledge that some factors are still missing. Vitamin B_6 relieves and improves conditions that are frequently associated with myocardial infarction, but this is as close as the vitamin comes to treatment and prevention of the heart attack. It is my opinion that a deficiency of vitamin B_6 is a primary factor involved in the development of diabetes and arteriosclerosis and that in association there is an imbalance of electrolytes—ionized magnesium, potassium, and calcium, in particular.

The American diet is already suspect as a cause of the high myocardial infarction rate. In this country we consume, on an average, 1.5 milligrams of vitamin B_6 daily, give or take 0.5 milligram. On the basis of my studies I would suggest that there is a dietary relationship between myocardial infarction and advanced vitamin B_6 deficiency. The "coronary prone" patient presents a clinical warning syndrome characterized by paresthesia of the hands, edema and reduced flexion of the fingers and hands, painful neuritis of the upper arms and shoulders, and nocturnal spasms of the feet and leg muscles—all of which can be, and have been, relieved by 50 milligrams of pyridoxine daily.

One has only to know that rheumatism and the shoulder-hand syndrome are responsive to vitamin B_6 to conclude that, somewhere between the early life of the fetus and the terminal gasps of the coronary-thrombosis victim, an increased need for vitamin B_6 stands paramount as an associate in the cause of the deadly heart attack, myocardial infarction.

When Laboratory and Clinic Agree II

"Every amino acid studied requires vitamin B_6 for its degradation."

Dr. Esmond E. Snell, the biochemist who discovered the pyridoxal and pyridoxamine forms of B_6, stated this in 1969 at the New York Academy of Sciences Symposium on vitamin B_6.[1] Vitamin B_6, then, is the "protein vitamin." Protein is made up of complex amino acids. When there is an insufficient supply of B_6, a chain of adverse chemical reactions takes place. The nutrient is necessary for protein metabolism in millions of human body cells. It enters into more than thirty enzymatic reactions, reported biochemist Henry Borsook of the Kerckhoff Biological Laboratories at the California Institute of Technology.[2] H. E. Sauberlich has since reported more than fifty enzymatic reactions in which B_6 participates.[3] These involve the cells in the brain, liver, blood, nerves, blood vessels, kidneys, muscles, and endocrine, or ductless, glands that produce certain hormones. As W. H. Sebrell, Jr., has suggested, "The fundamental metabolic role of vitamin B_6 is probably one of the reasons it is so widespread in nature."[4]

In the preceding chapters case after case has been presented of the clinical evidence of B_6 deficiency and its treatment. But what of other investigations in other clinics? Especially, what proof has come from the laboratories to support these clinical findings?

This chapter will seek to correlate experiments and studies, as reported by other scientists, with the work I have already described with my patients. In order to make it easier to comprehend, this chapter will follow, as far as possible, the organization of the preceding pages of this book.

HUMAN REQUIREMENTS FOR B₆

Until relatively recently, little was known regarding the results of vitamin B_6 deficiency in the human being, although researchers have extensively investigated the dietary requirements for the vitamin in poultry, swine, dogs, monkeys, rabbits, fox, mink, fish, ruminants,[5] and other animals.[6]

Some of the most extensive work with human beings in the laboratory has been accomplished with human volunteers at the U. S. Army Medical Research and Nutrition Laboratory at Denver, Colorado. Army researcher Howerde E. Sauberlich, Ph.D., one of the world authorities on B_6 in the laboratory, Colonel J. E. Canham, and their associates reported the results of their twelve-year project during the 1969 symposium of the New York Academy of Sciences.

Their volunteers consisted of young adult male soldiers who were housed and maintained on a metabolic ward where the dietary intake was rigidly controlled and their activity was constantly supervised. Multiple studies were conducted, some of which are of especial pertinence to this chapter. For instance, in one study, six subjects were fed a B_6-deficient, high-protein diet of 100 grams of protein daily. Electroencephalograms (EEG) were taken of their brain waves. Among these six, xanthurenic acid (XA) excretion did not rise markedly until after two weeks of depletion. By the end of the third week a point of acknowledged deficiency was reached—and five of the six had abnormal EEGs. At this point their diets were then supplemented with B_6, but during this subsequent period there was a delay in a return to normal of some of the EEGs. (The one subject whose EEG was normal throughout the study also paradoxically demonstrated the highest net excretion of XA and 2-hydroxykynurenine, another metabolite of tryptophan, during the depletion period.)

In another study using the tryptophan load test to register metabolic changes in subjects on B$_6$-deficient, low-protein (30 grams daily) diets, the xanthurenic-acid excretion did not become elevated until the end of the third week—a bit longer than in the high-protein group. Despite the fact that the XA excretion mean net was relatively low after three weeks of depletion, four of the five subjects recorded abnormal EEGs at that stage. During the last two weeks of the study, two grams of DL-methionine, another amino acid, was added to the formula diet—which apparently resulted directly in the rise of net XA excretion for those two weeks. (As in the previous group, the individual who had the highest net 3-hydroxykynurenine, 740 milligrams, and XA excretion, 405 milligrams, at the end also had normal EEGs throughout the study.) After six and a half weeks of depletion, one of the subjects required thirty days of regular diet, supplemented by 150 milligrams of pyridoxine daily, before he reverted to normal, as indicated by his EEGs.

Previously, in animal research reported in 1948, the laboratory had found that B$_6$ deficiencies were definitely made worse when methionine was added to the diet, thus indicating the vital role of B$_6$ in metabolizing this amino acid in particular.

The Army researchers were able to conclude that symptoms, in severity and rapidity of onset, related directly to the amount of protein in the diet. Furthermore, the requirement for B$_6$ seemed to be related directly to the protein intake. In some of the studies they were also to observe that "partial adaptation occurs in the human required to subsist on a submarginal intake of vitamin B$_6$," a factor complicating their accurately assessing the minimal requirement for human beings.

In an attempt to determine human requirements, as indicated in these young, healthy soldiers, the researchers showed that 30 grams of protein daily necessitated slightly more than 1 milligram of B$_6$, while those consuming 165 grams of protein per day seemed to need more than 1.93 milligrams.[7]

(Dr. Sauberlich and Colonel Canham, through studies of urinary metabolites and electroencephalograms, demonstrated this time relation of three to six weeks in producing changes with a B$_6$-

deficient diet or in correcting changes with vitamin B₆. This time factor of three to six weeks corresponds with my clinical findings that pain and paresthesia of rheumatism were relieved by B₆ within three to six weeks.)

However accurately these tests may have established the B₆ needs of these young soldiers at Ft. Simmons General Hospital in Colorado, it is obvious, from my work as well as that of others, that many persons require much more B₆ for various reasons. We have seen how some pregnant patients required hundreds of milligrams to relieve their signs and symptoms. W. H. Sebrell, Jr., M.D., of Columbia University's Institute of Nutrition Sciences, has pointed out that "the full clinical effect of the deficiency [of B₆] has not been determined for different ages or conditions of stress." And he added, "The weight of the evidence indicates to me that figures generally used are probably too low to be entirely safe for a large population group subject to a variety of stress situation." The effects of "long continued partial deficiency" also remain unknown, he stated.[8]

MENSTRUATION AND MENOPAUSE

All hormones are composed of complicated chains of amino acids. Because of this, and because of B₆'s being the "protein vitamin," one is probably safe in assuming that B₆ is essential, generally, to all hormone metabolism, as a result of numerous different complex biochemical reactions, both known and unknown.

When in the course of my clinical work I related B₆ deficiency with pregnancy, premenstrual edema, the menopause and menopausal symptoms, I knew, in my own mind, that pyridoxine was related to female hormone metabolism, but I did not know which hormone was involved. In 1969 I attended the New York Academy of Sciences symposium on "Vitamin B₆ in Metabolism of the Nervous System," where I heard a paper read by Dr. Merle Mason of the University of Michigan department of biological chemistry. I asked Dr. Mason to have lunch with me so I could discuss this problem with him. At that time he explained the female hormonal association with B₆ and suggested that I talk also with Dr. R. R.

Brown from the division of clinical oncology at the University of Wisconsin Medical School. Both Mason and Brown, on the basis of their extensive laboratory findings, assured me that an increased supply of estrogen in women taking the birth-control pills was requiring increased amounts of B_6.

In his paper at the symposium, Mason reported experiments conducted by him and his colleagues on the role of sex hormones. Several previous studies by other researchers had already indicated that injections of high levels of pyridoxine cause great increases in enzyme levels and that steroids, such as the sex hormones, may interfere with the actions of dietary factors. For instance, it had been shown that a decline in enzyme activity occurred more rapidly in animals that were treated with the B_6 antagonist deoxypyridoxine *and* testosterone, a so-called male hormone, than in those treated with deoxypyridoxine alone. Accordingly, Mason *et al.* set up an experiment to determine if ovarian hormones were responsible for the sex differences. The ovaries were removed from female rats. Months later an assay of the activities of the enzyme kynurenine transaminase was conducted. Ovariectomy in each case had resulted in a substantially higher enzyme level in the kidney tissue; in liver tissue there was no such change. The role of the ovaries in sex and enzyme differences had been demonstrated. Further experiments with rats showed the enzyme levels and other values of estrogen-treated males to be remarkably similar to those of normal females.

The evidence of the experiments demonstrated that steroid and non-steroid metabolites could cause a redistribution of pyridoxal phosphate (PLP) between apoenzymes. An apoenzyme is the purely protein part of an enzyme that, with the coenzyme, forms the complete or holenzyme. The researchers put forth the possibility that similar metabolic actions might account for "the ability of estrogens to cause changes in tryptophan metabolism resembling those occurring during pyridoxine deficiency."[9]

In careful, detailed laboratory work with rats, they had shown why women, because of their hormonal differences, may have medical complications that would require increased levels of vitamin B_6. Hormonal change and imbalances are particularly significant prior and during menstruation and at the time of menopause. As seen in Chapter 5, many women at these times do experience medical conditions that respond to B_6.

THE BIRTH-CONTROL PILL

By 1966 when my autobiographical book *The Doctor Who Looked at Hands* was published I had already concluded that there was an increased need for vitamin B_6 during pregnancy, during menopause, and during use of birth-control pills. Exactly what was happening was not clear, but it appeared that estrogen either required increased amounts of B_6 for its metabolic role or else it became toxic when there was insufficient B_6. Since the publication of my findings in 1966, a body of striking research with B_6 has been done by others in this area. The role of vitamin B_6 with the female hormone has been nailed down. When it was proved that increased female hormone supply and birth-control pills caused changes in the urinary metabolites and that these changes could be corrected by doses of up to 30 milligrams of pyridoxine daily, pyridoxine had then been linked to hormone oversupply. Thus, a need for increased pyridoxine was associated with an increased amount of the hormone.

A neat, perfect dovetail of proof has been constructed from the laboratory findings that support clinical experience. Among the earliest work was that of David P. Rose of the Department of Clinical Pathology at the University of Sheffield in Great Britain. (Dr. Rose later came to the University of Wisconsin.) Administering the tryptophan load test to fourteen women who had been taking various oral contraceptives, Rose discovered they excreted "grossly increased amounts of xanthurenic acid" in their urine. Then after five days' treatment with 40 milligrams of pyridoxine hydrochloride the fourteen women were retested for xanthurenic acid in the urine, and it had fallen from 593 milligrams to 80 milligrams in an eight-hour collection of urine. B_6 had made a dramatic change, and Rose proposed, "The marked fall in the excretion of xanthurenic acid by the subject treated with pyridoxine suggests that the hormonal effect may result from interference with the coenzyme function of pyridoxal-5-phosphate."[10]

In an extension of the early work by Rose, in relation to birth-control pills, J. M. Price and colleagues at the University of Wisconsin Medical School tested ten subjects with the tryptophan load test. An elevated excretion of xanthurenic acid occurred. They were then given 100 milligrams of pyridoxine daily. The tryptophan metabolism became normal, thus apparently demonstrating "another metabolic interrelationship between steroid hormones and pyridoxine."[11]

At Guy's Hospital Medical School in London, researchers P. A. Toseland and Sarah Price reported finding high levels of 3-hydroxyanthranilic acid (3HA) without tryptophan loading in two women taking oral contraceptives, as well as "significantly raised levels" in two other women. 3HA is a tryptophan metabolite and is a necessary precursor of nicotinic acid, another factor in the B complex. The study showed that 3HA rose in proportion to the length of time that the subject had been taking estrogen-progestogen compounds and that pyridoxine apparently reversed the increase of 3HA in the urine.[12] Subsequently, other researchers concluded that it was estrogen in the anovulatory drugs that caused the increased excretion of tryptophan metabolites. This was observed to be true in both men and women. The men studied were those with both benign and malignant prostate growth that were treated with estrogens.[13]

In a 1971 report by A. Leonard Luhby, M.D., and associates, a study conducted at the New York Medical College related urinary excretions after a tryptophan load test to oral doses of 2, 5, 10, and 20 milligrams of pyridoxine in women using oral contraceptives. The detrimental effects of various tryptophan metabolites were pointed out, including interference with glycogen manufacture (glyconeogenesis), insulin metabolism, oxidative phosphyrylation (a process in sugar metabolism), and in being carcinogenic, or cancer-causing. However, the 2-milligram dose of B₆ seemed to correct only 10 percent of the women studied; nor did the 20-milligram dose correct all of the subjects. It was revealed that 25 milligrams were needed to correct the tryptophan metabolism of all women on the Pill, and a dose of 30 milligrams daily was recommended. The researchers noted that from seven to eight million women were using birth-control pills in the United States alone.[14]

PREGNANCY

In the early nineteen forties, articles in the *American Journal of Obstetrics and Gynecology* had pointed out the importance of pyridoxine in preventing disturbances of early pregnancy. In 1951 Herbert Sprince and associates reported the investigation of five categories of female subjects and their urinary excretion of xanthurenic acid. The groups were of normal non-pregnant women, normal pregnant women (early last trimester), pre-eclamptic patients, eclamptic patients, and women in the last trimester of "normal" pregnancy with complications due to a concurrent disease. The investigators found a highly increased excretion of xanthurenic acid after a tryptophan load in the eclamptic and pre-eclamptic patients; the values for those two categories were similar. "In normal pregnant women, only a slight rise was noted, whereas normal nonpregnant women exhibited no change at all," they observed, noting that the xanthurenic excretion test might be "of value in the early detection of pre-eclampsia and eclampsia." They added: "It is possible that a deranged protein metabolism known to occur in such conditions may increase the metabolic demand for vitamin B_6 far beyond the normal optimal level of intake."[15] This is exactly what I have found to be true in the clinic.

Dr. Max Wachstein, pathologist at St. Catherine's Hospital in New York, very carefully documented the fact that a disturbance occurs in the metabolism of B_6 during pregnancy. In one series Wachstein administered test doses of 10 grams of tryptophan to normal patients as well as those ill with various diseases and those pregnant. Only small amounts of xanthurenic acid were found in the urine of the normal subjects and those who were ill. The pregnant women excreted increased amounts of xanthurenic acid. Wachstein found that xanthurenic-acid excretion began to increase at the end of the first trimester in the women's pregnancies. When pyridoxine was given, the high levels of the abnormal metabolite were reduced—in every instance. He noted that a substantial decrease in xanthurenic acid came after only three daily treatments with 25 milligrams of B_6. In three more days of pyridoxine treatment, the xanthurenic-acid level was as low as in the normal non-pregnant control patients.[16] Years later, Wachstein, then at Beth Israel Hospital in Passaic, New Jersey, was to conclude, "In pregnancy there is considerable evidence to support the assumption that the growing fetus draws vitamin B$_6$ from the maternal store since the cord blood contains much more total vitamin B$_6$, as well as the coenzymatically active pyridoxal phosphate, than does the maternal blood. The blood levels of pyridoxal phosphate and pyridoxamine phosphate furthermore are smaller in pregnant women at term than in nonpregnant controls."[17]

In Canada, Dr. Sidney M. Tobin at the New Mt. Sinai Hospital in Toronto reported that 50 percent of the obstetricians responding to a questionnaire had found numbness and tingling to be a common complaint in pregnancy. But only 15 percent, he noted, sought any further details from the patient, and only one out of every ten obstetricians considered the carpal tunnel syndrome in diagnosing the paresthesia. The rest of them considered it of circulatory nature or a metabolic change due to pregnancy. In this 1967 report the carpal tunnel mystery remained unsolved.[18] As seen in Chapters 4 and 7, the carpal tunnel syndrome as well as other signs and symptoms associated with pregnancy have responded to vitamin B$_6$.

Toxemia remains the gravest single danger of pregnancy, as discussed in Chapter 7. Drs. Jack A. Klieger, Charles H. Altshuler, and associates at St. Joseph's Hospital in Milwaukee have shown that toxic placentas are "markedly deficient in pyridoxine when compared to the normal placentas." They have shown that extracts from toxic placentas have an average of 0.34 micrograms of pyridoxal phosphate per milligram of protein, while normal placentas have an average of 0.86 micrograms, more than twice as much. They also have suggested that the tryptophan load test, which tests for xanthurenic acid, may not be accurate or may be too simplistic. Pointing out that the quantity of tryptophan used is important, they suggest that sometimes too much may be used and produce unrealisic test results. Furthermore, more than xanthurenic-acid tests may be needed to gauge B$_6$ deficiency, especially the evaluation of both 3-hydroxykynurenic and 3-hydroxyanthranilic acid, which "is now considered to reflect more accurately the vitamin B$_6$ status of the patient."[19]

As was demonstrated in Chapter 7, toxemic patients have been treated successfully in the clinic with vitamin B_6. An association of the carpal tunnel syndrome with pregnancy has been established, and it has been clearly demonstrated that laboratory data and therapy with pyridoxine are in perfect agreement.

LIFE IN UTERO AND AFTERWARD

In Chapter 8 were shown clinical results of B_6 therapy in the infant and the child. One will recall the instances in which the edematous mother was treated with B_6 and experienced dramatic reduction of swelling, a relatively short time before delivery, and consequently the baby was born with wrinkled skin. The wrinkling of the newborn's skin was interpreted as meaning that the baby had been edematous *in utero* and had, like the mother, gained relief from the swelling as a direct result of the B_6. Cases were also presented in Chapter 8 of small children who were treated with B_6.

Fortunately, other investigators in other hospitals have compiled laboratory data that clearly support my own clinical findings. One of the earliest, most perceptive of investigators in this field has been Dr. David Baird Coursin of the Research Institute at St. Joseph Hospital in Lancaster, Pennsylvania. By using the electroencephalogram (EEG) with patients, he was able to record objectively the changes in brain waves as a result of B_6 insufficiency.

In one case of a B_6-dependent retarded child, Coursin maintained her on 10 milligrams of pyridoxine daily. Several times during a five-year period, vitamin B_6 was withdrawn from the patient on a trial basis, while she continued on her normal diet. "The elimination of her daily pyridoxine was tolerated quite well for the first 48 hours," reported Coursin. "She then began to show minimal signs of mental confusion, decreased coordination, some irritability, and transient periods of lapses of consciousness with open eyes and some staring. . . . By the end of 76 hours, these symptoms were much more noticeable." With published excerpts from her EEG, Coursin was able to indicate concretely what effects the withdrawal of B_6 had. At the end of 120 hours she was treated with intravenous pyridoxine. A total of 100 milligrams was administered in a forty-three-minute period, but her EEG had become normal thirty minutes after the injections had been started. In fact, within twelve minutes, after 20 milligrams of B_6, she had "well established changes in her EEG and was showing marked clinical improvement." By the following morning she was back to her usual self before the experiment and was continued thereafter on 10 milligrams of pyridoxine daily.

Based on his observations and laboratory data, as well as work of other scientists, Coursin was able to suggest that "the detrimental effects of pyridoxine dependency may become operant *in utero* at a critical time during parturition." Outlining central nervous system disorders in which B_6 may have a role, he listed epilepsy, convulsive seizures, mental retardation, phenylpyruvic oligophrenia, and mongolism. He indicated the risks of convulsive seizures and mental retardation in the infant receiving an inadequate supply of B_6. He also called attention to those infants whose B_6 deficiency might go undetected when he stated: "It also appears highly probable that a far greater number will have molecular changes in intracellular metabolism without obvious clinical symptoms. Over prolonged periods (perhaps years) of ingestion of a diet with marginal B_6, there may be physiological adaptation of the individual so that biochemical alterations may continue without disturbing clinical signs but with some limitation in general growth and CNS capacity."[20]

Coursin had shown the remarkable effect of a B_6 injection on a patient having convulsions. Following the injection the patient's brain-wave forms improved and rapidly become normal. As Coursin said, "The major contribution of these observations lay in the fact that they served as an unequivocal demonstration of the effect of a single nutrient on brain function—linking the neurochemical, neurophysiological and clinical performance patterns." The individual differences, however, undoubtedly would be significant, he said, so that the requirements for a few individuals will be higher than the estimates for the normal population. For some patients, small amounts of pyridoxine will be sufficient to reverse their symptoms; others will require large amounts "to balance the heritable alteration in binding properties of a specific apoenzyme requiring pyridoxal phosphate for normal activity. . . . The usual normal levels of B_6 in the diet and in tissues are not sufficient for the requirements of these individuals, so that their abnormally higher requirement for the vitamin results in a state of subcellular B_6 deficiency."[21]

On children, as noted earlier in adults, the conventional tryptophan load test has been questioned. Olle Hansson of the Uppsala, Sweden, University Hospital's department of pediatrics, among others, has pointed out its limitations in precisely measuring B_6 deficiency.[22] That is not to say, of course, that the tryptophan load test has not been extremely helpful, for without it many associations with B_6 deficiency would have been overlooked.

Malnutrition has long been recognized as a threat to the pregnant woman and her fetus. Research has now pinpointed some of the specific risks that face the fetus-baby before and after birth. D. N. Raine of the biochemistry department at Children's Hospital at Birmingham, England, has pointed out that "the onset of infantile spasms is often within the first year of life but only rarely before three months of age." He has correlated this with previous reports that the pyridoxine level in the brain starts to increase approximately in the second month of life. "It is at this period that both myelination and growth are especially active, and it is possible that if such an increased demand for pyridoxine is not met, permanent damage may result."[23] Myelination refers to the forming of myelin, which is the white, fatty substance that makes a sheath around certain nerve fibers. An infant's brain is still developing in the first several months after birth. Brain tissues must have pyridoxine or suffer irreversible damage. The stakes are too high to neglect what has already been proved—that overnutrition of the infant with B_6 is far better than the risks of undernutrition with B_6.

Experiments with rats have left no doubt as to the dangers of a B_6-deficient environment *in utero*. Three investigators at the University of Washington School of Medicine's department of pediatrics—Starkey D. Davis, Thomas Nelson, and Thomas H. Shepard—demonstrated birth defects in experiments with B_6-deficient rats.[24] Using a deficient diet and a specific B_6 antagonist, 4-deoxypyridoxine, they induced B_6 deficiency in pregnant rats and studied the results.

The mother rats developed skin changes typical of B_6 deficiency. On the twentieth day the pregnant does of both the treated group and the untreated control group were killed and their fetuses examined. The B_6-deficient fetuses were small and many of them appeared edematous, conditions directly attributable to the diet. Defects were found in their abdomens, ranging from mild defects of viscera protruding through abdominal defects to severe defects involving major portions of the liver, stomach, pancreas, spleen, the small intestine, and part of the colon.

Gross defects were found in the extremities of the B_6-deficient fetuses as against *none* in the control group. Of the 108 live fetuses in the test group, forty-eight had digital defects, twenty had cleft palate, and twenty-six had other gross defects. And based on their experiment and the work of previous investigators, they added: "We anticipate that fetal B_6 deficiency will cause a permanent immunologic defect."

Not only did this experiment establish that vitamin B_6 deficiencies can lead to birth defects, as it did in the test rats, but it also linked the deficiency to defects in immunologic, neurologic, and skeletal makeup. The edematous fetuses also help document my own clinical experiences in which I found wrinkled skin on babies whose mothers' edema had been reduced in the ninth month of pregnancy by large doses of B_6. I had presumed that the babies were edematous *in utero;* the experiments with the B_6-deficient rats proved that such fetuses *are* edematous.

In related work, Oswald Wiss and Fritz Weber of the Hoffmann-La Roche Company research department have shown that when mother rats were put on B_6-free diets immediately after giving birth, "about 50% of the young rats showed cerebral symptoms, often with seizures, even after as short a period as 2–3 weeks."[25] The relationship of pyridoxine to immunology has been documented by A. E. Axelrod and Anthony C. Trakatellis of the University of Pittsburgh School of Medicine.[26]

The role of nutritional deficiency in causing birth defects had been well established as long ago as 1932 when Fred Hale, at the Texas Agricultural Experiment Station at College Station, Texas, produced birth defects in piglets farrowed of a sow on a vitamin A-deficient diet. Eleven pigs were born; all of them were born without eyeballs.[27] In subsequent experiments Hale got the same results, with blind pigs born to gilts on vitamin A-deficient diets; on the other hand, gilts given small amounts of cod-liver oil during gestation period farrowed normal litters.[28]

In all, by 1935, Hale had reported four litters of forty-two pigs born blind in his experiments. Other birth defects noted included cleft palate, cleft lip, accessory ears, and kidney defects. Hereditary factors were ruled out after careful investigation; the defects were ascribed to vitamin A deficiencies alone. "Vitamin-A deficiency is by no means uncommon in human diet and it may easily be that many of the eye weaknesses which we suffer today are due to maternal vitamin-A deficiency," wrote Hale. And he added: "We should insist on an abundance of vitamin A in the diet of the expectant mother in the early stages of pregnancy when so many of the vital organs of the embryo are being formed."[29] In documenting the experiments Hale also reported one gilt that had received a single dose of cod-liver oil two weeks before conception; she subsequently gave birth to pigs with eyes, but they were blind and had other defects. Thus he was able to demonstrate that the severity of birth defects was in direct proportion to the degree of dietary deficiency of vitamin A.[30]

Hale's work paved the way for subsequent work on nutritional causes of birth defects by establishing that a key vitamin such as vitamin A was so important in fetal life. Now that B_6-deficient mother rats have produced offspring with birth defects, it might be pointed out that the obtaining of sufficient B_6 for the mother during pregnancy is probably much more difficult than her receiving an adequate level of vitamin A. The usual American diet has less vitamin B_6 than it has vitamin A.

In 1972 I visited with the brothers Drs. Louis Greenberg and David Greenberg at the University of California School of Medicine at San Francisco. Dr. David Greenberg, the biochemist, had worked with a factor that is important in causing mental retardation. He isolated the pyridoxal phosphate-catalyzed enzyme system that breaks down cystathionine to cysteine and homoserine in the brain. He told me then, "A child may be mentally retarded because there is an accumulation of cystathionine in the brain." In effect, then, one form of mental retardation is caused by a metabolic malfunction related to an amino acid in the brain. Vitamin B$_6$ is necessary for the utilization of that particular amino acid—in this instance, methionine.

In that same discussion, Dr. Louis Greenberg, the pathologist, commented that in persons with an inborn error of blood-cell development in which there is anemia, approximately 100 milligrams of pyridoxine are required daily to sustain a normal red-blood-cell count.

During that same trip I also visited Dr. Esmond E. Snell at the University of California at Berkeley. In discussing my work in northeast Texas he asked me how long it took for a recurrence of symptoms, such as paresthesia in the hands, on discontinuation of B$_6$ therapy.

"Three to six weeks," I replied.

He said, "These people must have a high requirement for vitamin B$_6$."

After spending two afternoons with these scientists at the University of California at Berkeley and the University of California School of Medicine at San Francisco, there was no doubt in my mind—and I think there was none in their minds—that an increased need for vitamin B$_6$ can affect so many enzymatic reactions that the associated clinical symptomatology will be bizarre and difficult to evaluate and may be manifest in many different organs and systems of the body. Certainly it was my conclusion that since B$_6$ deficiency could cause disease in the brain, especially mental retardation, it becomes mandatory that we protect other systems against deficiency. This means that when any sign or symptom of increased need occurs, we must insure that the B$_6$ supply is more than adequate.

DIABETES

A biochemist for one of the leading laboratories in this country has told me, "Nobody knows how insulin works." A few enzymatic exchanges are understood. After that there is a great wasteland of ignorance, although there are very reasonable theories. A leading textbook in biochemistry states it thusly: "Despite complete elucidation of the structure of insulin, there is still no understanding of the relationship between the structure of the protein and its biological action."[31] As the authors explain, diabetes mellitus is produced by insulin deficiency and a consequent failure by certain tissues to utilize glucose. The precise mechanism that brings this about is less clear. For example, diabetes can be caused by an oversecretion of more than one hormone from more than one endocrine gland. The pancreas, in other words, may not necessarily be the only endocrine gland involved, and insulin may not be the only hormone. Hypothetically, if a deficiency of B_6 is associated with hormone metabolism, then B_6 deficiency could be a cause of diabetes.

Yakito Kotake of Japan's Wakayama Medical College has demonstrated that xanthurenic acid is capable of causing diabetes in animals.[32] Although the scientific community has not accepted with open arms Kotake's concept that increased xanthurenic acid causes diabetes in humans, his studies undeniably proved that diabetes could be regularly produced in albino rats with diets high in fat, high in the protein tryptophan, and low in vitamin B_6. This experimental diet also simultaneously produced an excess of xanthurenic acid.

Since human diabetes is of a chronic nature, Kotake and his associates also studied the role of xanthurenic acid in the development of chronic diabetic symptoms. He continued the rats on the high-fat, high-tryptophan diet for 240 days. Xanthurenic-acid excretion continued high. On about the 170th day, after regular and steady weight gains, they grew obese and blood sugar levels also became elevated, paralleling the body weight pattern.* In other experiments, in which 10 milligrams of tryptophan were added to the diet daily, the albino rats gradually gained weight for the first thirty days, then lost; on about the 100th day there was a marked drop, and during the period from the 230th to the 250th day they died. During this experiment a rapid increase in the blood sugar level became apparent on about the thirty-fifth day, parallel with B_6 deficiency, and thereafter the blood sugar level rose to 160 to 200 milligrams per 100 milliliters. Some of the rats had

* 170 to 200 milligrams per 100 milliliters, King and Garner's method.

true blood sugar levels of around 400 milligrams during the whole course of the experiment. Xanthurenic-acid excretion was recorded from the thirtieth day on, and it amounted to 4 to 7 milligrams daily—a high figure.

Kotake concluded that xanthurenic acid has an accumulative effect on the development of diabetes, which is in keeping with the fact that human diabetes usually progresses chronically.

Kotake also demonstrated, in a study of twenty-three diabetic patients in the Wakayama Medical College hospital, that "XA [xanthurenic acid] in a free form was invariably present in the urines of diabetic patients—the fact leads us to conclude that there is an undeniable etiological relation between free XA and human diabetes." It was Kotake's opinion that xanthurenic acid inhibits hexose phosphorylation and thus inhibits glucose metabolism, while helping to store glucose in the blood; this process therefore gives rise to diabetogenic symptoms as hyperglycemia (high blood sugar) and glucosura (glucose in the urine).

To me, Kotake's work is a milestone in the search for the causes of diabetes mellitus; he proved, in the laboratory, that a high-fat, high-protein diet—rich in tryptophan and low in B₆—will cause diabetes. To a large extent this is the American diet today, and it is the same diet maintained by many clinicians even after their patients have been diagnosed as being diabetic. The results have been little short of catastrophic.

Chapter 9 shows, beyond doubt, that the symptomatology of neuritis and neuropathies of the fingers and hands is worse in diabetics, and it is responsive to vitamin B₆.

Since diabetes is a notorious associate of arteriosclerosis, I asked Dr. Louis Greenberg in 1972 if he had found any association between the two during his research with monkeys. B₆-deficient diets had caused a type of arteriosclerosis in these experimental animals; I wondered if he had noted any diabetic signs. Dr. Greenberg informed me that the monkeys did not have elevated blood sugar levels as are found in diabetes mellitus. However, rats on B₆-deficient diets did have a change in the pancreas, he said. In 1958 he had reported, at the International Academy of Biochemistry meeting in Moscow, that the pancreases of rats on B₆-deficient diets, above all other tissues, showed the highest transulfuration activity. This meant, in effect, that there was laboratory evidence that B_6 deficiency was altering the biochemical exchanges in the pancreas.

Among the interesting laboratory work pertaining to diabetes, and possibly to hypoglycemia, is that of Gerold M. Grodsky and Leslie L. Bennett, reported in 1966. Extracting a rat pancreas and isolating it in a perfusion tube in which solutions could flow through, they introduced glucose into the perfused rat pancreas and produced a graded insulin response within thirty seconds after glucose entry. Furthermore, the response ended within thirty seconds after the glucose's disappearance from their glucose "pulse" experiments. The experiment demonstrated that a glucose-stimulated pancreas has no "memory" but secretes insulin only during stimulation.

Grodsky and Bennett further showed that glucagon, another hormone secreted by the pancreas, stimulated insulin secretion directly, in the absence of glucose. Although this indicates that insulin secretion is sensitively controlled by glucose concentration, other substances such as glucagon, calcium, and potassium may act at more primary sites in the release mechanism, independently of glucose concentration, to become controlling factors in patients with diabetes, pancreatic tumors, or aldosteronism. (Aldosteronism, or an excess of this powerful adrenal hormone, is associated with hypertension.) Calcium, for instance, is required for insulin secretion; in its absence, the tissue remained viable, but glucose stimulation of insulin secretion was totally blocked. By adding calcium twenty to forty minutes later, the blockage was reversed and insulin secreted. Potassium, raised to 8 milliequivalents per liter, was a direct stimulant of insulin release in the absence of glucose.[33]

In other experiments Bennett, Grodsky, and Donald L. Curry demonstrated that magnesium and calcium are competitive for the same active site at the cell membrane or at the granule membrane. They found that "when sites are bound by magnesium ion, calcium ion cannot exert its permissive or facilitating effect on secretion" of insulin. The experiments, reported in *Endocrinology,* showed that when magnesium concentration was two or three times greater than calcium, "complete inhibition of secretion [of insulin] occurred."

They ran five series of experiments, with the same amount of glucose used in each case. In Series No. 1, calcium was used without magnesium; insulin was secreted in all instances. In No. 2, with equal portions of calcium and magnesium, half secreted insulin, half did not. In No. 3, magnesium was doubled over that of calcium and there was "essentially complete inhibition of insulin secretion." In No. 4, calcium was raised to the level of magnesium used in Series No. 3, so that calcium and magnesium were equal, and the pancreases secreted insulin. In Series No. 5, again insulin secretion was blocked when the magnesium level doubled that of calcium, which in turn was overcome by raising the calcium to an equal level; but when magnesium was elevated three times the level of calcium, none of the preparations secreted insulin.[34]

Other experiments relating to insulin were done at the University of New Mexico School of Medicine by R. Whang, R. Wagner, and D. Rodgers in which they concluded that both serum potassium and magnesium can be decreased by glucose and insulin infusion. Two groups of subjects intravenously received one liter of 5 percent dextrose in water. Group 1, with seven patients, had ten units of regular insulin; Group 2, with eight patients, had fifteen units. Group 1 "exhibited no statistically significant changes." Group 2 patients "were found to have small but statistically significant decreases" in serum potassium, magnesium, and phosphate.[35] As they pointed out, previous studies by others had indicated that insulin promotes the cellular influx of both potassium and magnesium.

The clinical significance of these experiments becomes clearer when one returns to two patients in previous chapters—S. S. in Chapter 7, who had eclampsia during pregnancy, and N. H. in Chapter 9, who had a bowel obstruction. Each had convulsions; each also had diabetes mellitus. There is a loose relationship between vitamin B₆ dependency or deficiency and convulsions, and there is a definite relationship between B₆, magnesium, and several enzymatic reactions. The pregnant patient S. S. convulsed after receiving large doses of the hormone oxytocin and lactated Ringer's solution; afterward convulsions subsided to a degree. But she convulsed again after receiving a dose of insulin. N. H., the diabetic with bowel obstruction, had been vomiting all day, thereby losing her magnesium, and she presented convulsions that, according to the medical literature, are characteristic of magnesium deficiency.[36] When the lactated Ringer's solution was discontinued, convulsions subsided within sixty seconds. Magnesium supplementation, then, wasn't sufficient alone; something in the lactated Ringer's solution, probably calcium, had to be withdrawn also. *Both of these patients also convulsed after insulin injection,* and in both there was probably a relative magnesium deficit, the result of electrolyte imbalance.

Returning to the experiments with the perfused rat pancreas: it will be remembered that insulin is not secreted when the magnesium level is greater than the calcium level. There must be a balance for the two metallic ions to assist the pancreas properly in its role of blood sugar regulation. But on the basis of these clinical observations and the laboratory work discussed here, it would appear that large doses of magnesium sulfate will control eclampsia by controlling the output of insulin in an individual who is hypersensitive to insulin, when there is an electrolyte imbalance.

From what I have learned with these two diabetic patients, S. S. and N. H., I would say that insulin is the driving force that changes and moves these electrolytes, especially magnesium. But while magnesium is not readily excreted, potassium is lost in great quantities daily in the urine, a fact that makes a high intake of potassium-rich foods essential. Yet, it has been proved, as will be seen subsequently, that serum magnesium is low in the diabetic, possibly because of insulin reaction and frequent urination. For this reason, magnesium supplementation is needed in treatment of diabetes and more especially in the diabetic pregnant patients.

My evaluation of diabetic patients under various forms of physiological stress has led me to the opinion that, regardless of blood sugar levels, high or low, patients with a long-standing need for vitamin B_6 are hypersensitive to insulin. This hypersensitivity, more acute when calcium is high and magnesium is low, is best controlled by stabilizing insulin secretion by dietary measures— which, in addition to sugar regulation, include supplements of the two co-factors, pyridoxine and magnesium.

MAGNESIUM

Although magnesium is far greater in volume in the human body than is B$_6$, the two are co-factors in several enzymatic reactions. In an effort to explain more clearly the very complicated biochemical reactions that involve magnesium and pyridoxine, I asked my friend Dr. Maria C. Linder, of the Massachusetts Institute of Technology Department of Biochemistry, to give her view of these reactions, especially for this book.

"In the body," said Dr. Linder, "vitamin B$_6$ and magnesium are found attached to many enzymes and are essential for the function of these enzymes as catalysts in metabolism. The actions of vitamin B$_6$ are important primarily in one area of metabolism, namely the formation and utilization of amino acids. Amino acids are the building blocks for construction of the proteins of the body but can also be used as a source of energy when this is required. Magnesium, on the other hand, is active in all areas of metabolism wherever energy-producing or energy-requiring reactions are taking place. Thus it plays a role both in the burning of sugar to produce energy and in the utilization of this energy to produce body substances."[37]

One of the most extensive studies of magnesium in human metabolism is the one made at the Dartmouth Medical School and Brattleboro Memorial Hospital in Vermont by Dr. Henry Schroeder and associates. They studied magnesium in human tissue and its sources in food, water, and air. Samples of human tissues were obtained frozen, then ashed in muffle furnaces and analyzed by emission spectroscopy. In all they used 399 subjects, including 197 U.S. subjects and 202 subjects from foreign lands. They arrived at magnesium statistics for what they considered a "standard man."

In this "standard man," 55 percent of the total magnesium was in bone, 26.5 percent in muscle, and the lowest level in fat. There was more magnesium than calcium in muscle, about 150 percent that of calcium in the soft tissues, although the total body content was only 2 percent that of calcium. The highest concentration of magnesium was found in the larynx and in the aorta, which also contain much calcium. The large intestine had more magnesium than did the upper gastrointestinal tract.

Magnesium acts as a bridge in a large number of chemical reactions that result in transfers of organic groups from one molecule to another. When organic phosphate takes part in a reaction, magnesium is usually with the inorganic factor, and magnesium apparently does not take part in any mammalian reaction where phosphate is not involved. Ingested magnesium is absorbed mainly by the small intestine. Because calcium and magnesium probably have common absorptive sites, calcium may compete with magnesium partly to inhibit the absorption of magnesium when calcium is present in large amounts. The serum magnesium levels remain remarkably constant in healthy persons.

In order for one to achieve daily equilibrium one needs 6 milligrams of magnesium per kilogram of body weight. This amounts to 420 milligrams for a 70-kilogram man. A daily intake of less than this may result in a negative balance. Schroeder *et al.* consider this daily intake absolutely necessary in order to insure good health. "To conclude that a negative balance of any major essential element exists throughout life is unrealistic and inconsistent with health and survival." But cases of deficiency are slow in appearing even under extreme conditions, and they may be relieved by an injection of 240 milligrams of magnesium intravenously. Magnesium doesn't store up in fat (if it did, it might throw off the body weight formula); in healthy persons, any magnesium in the urine over 12 milligrams per day represents an excess that is not required by the body.[38]

Citing the findings of previous investigators, they found that, under extreme conditions, sweating could account for 25 percent of the magnesium lost daily—a significant figure when one's intakes are low. They also pointed out the laboratory documentation on the negative features of diuretics, showing how the excessive use of diuretics can lead to depletion of magnesium as well as other minerals. William O. Smith and associates in an Oklahoma City study, among others, have documented the magnesium-depleting effects of diuretics in human volunteers.[39]

Laboratory support of my own clinical experience with hypomagnesemia (low blood magnesium) and diabetes, as seen particularly in the two patients S. S. and N. H., is shown by a study done in a private clinic in Indiana by Drs. Charles E. Jackson and Donald W. Meier. They drew 5,100 consecutive blood serums and found that diabetes mellitus was the disease condition most frequently found in association with low-serum magnesium.[40] Whether magnesium imbalance is a cause of diabetes or diabetes is a factor in hypomagnesemia, magnesium supplementation is obviously needed in these cases.

As for magnesium and eclampsia of pregnancy, Dr. C. E. Flowers, Jr., of the University of North Carolina School of Medicine has demonstrated, using magnesium sulfate, that serum magnesium levels of around 5 to 8 milligrams percent usually control convulsions until labor can be induced and the baby delivered. Flowers' report also suggested that large doses of morphine and barbiturates were unnecessary if there was sufficient magnesium.[41]

One gains further insight into human magnesium needs when one examines observations and research relating to these mineral imbalances in animals. Particularly pertinent data are available on cattle, on which my friend E. E. Neal, Jr., county agent for Titus County, Texas, has compiled a report especially for this book. Neal is a graduate of the School of Agriculture, Texas A & M University. In cattle, "grass tetany" is the usual term for low magnesium levels. Reported Neal:

Grass tetany is primarily a disease of older beef cattle and nursing cattle. The disease is not new, but occurs sporadically in various areas from coast to coast. The majority of cases occur while cows are grazing lush winter pastures although the disease may appear in starved cattle receiving only hay.

Grass tetany is sometimes called lactation tetany, grass staggers, wheat pasture poisoning or hypomagnesemia. Although the precise cause is unknown, it is usually associated with an imbalance in the mineral components of blood serum—particularly a low level of magnesium. The disease usually strikes before the forage has reached maturity and is usually associated with high fertilization rates, particularly potash. Serum calcium drops to 6.5-7.0 milligrams per cent and serum magnesium from a normal of 2.2-3.0 to below 1.0 milligrams per cent.

Most of the cases observed have been in lactating cows, two to eight weeks after calving. Cold, rainy weather is frequently present when the disease occurs. A combination of calving, weather, lactation, and other stress factors are thought to act as a triggering mechanism. Not only is the animal under stress, but the high protein content of young, tender grass produces a considerable amount of ammonia in the digestive tract, creating an alkaline situation which reduces the normal absorption of calcium and magnesium.

Soil and plants are usually normal in magnesium. With high fertilization rates, the potassium level in the plant may be increased. This high potassium level is competitive with magnesium; consequently, magnesium absorption is further reduced, resulting in an abnormal balance of electrolytes. Magnesium plays a vital role in energy metabolism and in the stability of the nervous system. Researchers have isolated a chemical, transaconitinic acid, from lush rye grass and wheat, which when fed to cattle along with large amounts of potassium produces grass tetany. The experimental disease is accompanied by lowered serum calcium and magnesium, and elevated serum potassium levels, just as in the clinical disease. Calcium content of the lush tender grass is also low.

Tetany symptoms include extreme nervousness, viciousness, trembling, staggering, falling, convulsions, and coma. Frequently the animal is found dead without these symptoms being observed. As you can see, this sporadic disease is difficult to predict or understand. Many herds of lactating cows have utilized winter pastures with no difficulty. More information is needed on soil types, amount of potash fertilizer applied, availability of soil magnesium, etc., as related to this disease.

The most reliable prevention is to be sure cows receive a large daily intake of magnesium oxide. In successful preventative programs, cattle have received from ½ to 2 ounces of pure magnesium oxide per head per day. No harmful effects have been observed when daily levels exceeded 6 ounces per day; evidently the excess is readily excreted.

In addition to his own observations Neal had also consulted experts in the field, including Steven S. Nicholson, associate specialist in veterinary science at Louisiana State University, and Dr. Randall Grooms, area livestock specialist of the Texas A & M University's Extension Service. But much of the data had come from Neal's personal experience as he dovetailed on-the-spot observations with laboratory results. His report continued:

We had a great deal of experience with this problem during an intensified grazing program on a prominent rancher's operation in Titus County [Texas], in the fall of 1970 and again in the fall of 1971. On this ranch there were 500 head of black Angus cows on 500 acres of pasture land. For five years, beginning in 1966, 350 pounds of 9-23-30 (nitrate-phosphate-potash formula) commercial fertilizer was added per acre to the soil each fall. In addition, 600 to 800 pounds per acre of ammonium nitrate was spread throughout the spring and summer. Also during this five-year period the land received two applications of lime.

In the fall of 1970 four cows died and in the fall of 1971 three cows died. Blood samples of two dead cows each year were sent to the diagnostic laboratory at Texas A & M University. Serum magnesium of the two animals in 1970 was recorded as 0.6 milligrams per cent and 0.3 milligrams per cent. In 1971 the two blood samples showed 0.2 milligrams per cent and 0.5 milligrams per cent. Although these blood levels for magnesium were low, soil and plant tests showed the magnesium content to be medium to high.

Immediately after we found the dead cows we gave the cattle on this particular ranch 100 pounds of magnesium oxide per ton of feed, and no more cows died. It was our overall conclusion that there was an imbalance between magnesium and potassium in the fertilization program. Regardless of what the precipitating factor or factors were, we were convinced that these animals were in dire need of magnesium supplements.[42]

The fertilization program for five years on this Texas ranch was very similar to the fertilization programs of vegetable growers in California, the Rio Grande Valley of Texas, and other rich agricultural areas of the United States. Thousands of refrigerated trucks and railroad cars carry these vegetables to distant cities each day. The scientific community must assume responsibility for preserving proper mineral balance in vegetables produced for our citizens.

Cows eating grass and hay are not necessarily so far removed from the human picture, for all of our food supply comes from the soil eventually, whether it is meat, vegetable, or fruit. Even fish may be affected by the mineral composition of their food. In fact, the magnesium levels of cows may be more significant to us than that of any other domesticated animal, for few animals are as controlled by the hand of man as the modern American cow. And cattle, with meat and milk, also make major contributions to the American diet.

The magnesium-calcium imbalance, which may be quite a serious problem for thousands of patients, is often made worse by the fact that cow's milk, a major constituent of the American diet, is a poor source of magnesium. Because it is high in calcium and low in magnesium, milk must be considered a food, not a whole food, in infant nutrition. Iron-deficiency anemia is very common in infants because other foods are not always given along with milk. Milk is also low in pyridoxine. Milk, for instance, has 11.5 milliequivalents of magnesium per kilogram, while meats, whole grains, raw green vegetables have more than 20 milliequivalents per kilogram.[43]

These facts provide irrefutable proof that the nursing mother needs to take magnesium supplements, not only for herself but especially for her baby's sake.

Keeping a sufficient supply of calcium is practically no problem at all, compared with that of magnesium. Most of the prenatal supplements supplied by pharmaceutical companies are high in calcium and low in magnesium. A low serum calcium level is so rare that one almost has to have a parathyroid abnormality to have such a calcium deficiency in the blood. The only instances of calcium tetany I have seen were in babies with severe diarrhea. Yet in spite of the body's mechanisms to guard against it, hypomagnesemia is relatively common. Because the kidney can conserve magnesium so well generally, the magnesium balance at the cell level is not readily changed. But over a period of time mild magnesium deficiency can occur because the patient does not eat the green plants that contain magnesium. This is particularly true of children.

The role of pure milk diets in causing magnesium deficiency is vividly illustrated by dairy experts who have proved that young calves fed as long as seventeen weeks on milk alone will spontaneously develop low blood magnesium tetany.[44] Even more graphic is the case of a human subject, the unusual case of a tetany syndrome in a woman excessively lactating. She had been lactating approximately 2,400 milliliters per day for three months. When a doctor first saw her she had painful cramping carpopedal spasms. Her blood calcium level was normal, 4.8 milliequivalents, but her magnesium level, at 0.4 milliequivalents, was low. She was given calcium intravenously, but the symptoms continued. But when she ceased lactating and got on a normal diet (which presumably was a sufficient source of magnesium), her symptoms were corrected as the serum magnesium concentration rose spontaneously to normal.[45]

In the clinic, muscle spasms in the legs, feet, arms, and hands provide the best evidence of mineral imbalance. The four horsemen of metallic exchange at the cell level are magnesium, calcium, sodium, and potassium. Magnesium and calcium, to a great extent, are locked inside the cells; their companion minerals, potassium and sodium, are outside the cells and active in exchanges. Muscle spasms that are indicative of deficiencies in vitamin B$_6$ and at least one of these minerals are common complaints in American clinics.

A brief example will illustrate my point. A woman, sixty-two, complained to me of painful cramps and spasms of the arms and hands, feet and legs. She had many of the same symptoms of numbness and tingling that so often had proved responsive to pyridoxine. Her fingers were painfully bowed at the metacarpophalangeal joints in both hands. Clinicians call this "carpal spasms." During flexion her finger joints popped and snapped, probably caused by the simultaneous pull of the tendons in extending and flexing the hands. She also had some terrible teeth; all of her lower incisors were decayed. Generally miserable for some time, she had suffered painful muscle spasms and had slept little over the past week. During the past two weeks she had been eating little but milk and soups.

While still in my office she was given two tablets that contained magnesium and potassium aspartate. By the time she reached her home in a taxicab her muscle spasms had subsided. The tablets contained a total of 500 milligrams of magnesium aspartate and 500 milligrams of potassium aspartate—about one half day's supply of each mineral, which she could have got from green vegetables if she had been able to eat them. She was given the magnesium and potassium tablets every six hours for forty-eight hours. She was relieved of spasms and pain. But her most valuable benefit may have been her improved sleep, for she was positive that her sound sleep thereafter was unusual and came as a result of the magnesium and potassium supplements.

One practical application seems clear. If a person cannot chew raw fruits and raw vegetables, he or she needs the juices of the raw vegetables. Dietitians, especially those who are employed in nursing homes where there are so many aged and debilitated persons, need to work diligently with delectable blends of juices from raw vegetables and raw fruits.

HEART DISEASE

In 1972, as mentioned, I spent an afternoon at the University of California School of Medicine in San Francisco with two brothers, Dr. Louis Greenberg, professor of pathology, and Dr. David Greenberg, professor of biochemistry. Louis Greenberg is one of the pioneers in research on the links between heart disease and B_6 deficiency. In 1949 he and Dr. J. F. Rinehart published their paper in the *American Journal of Pathology* on arteriosclerosis in monkeys fed a B_6-deficient diet. Twenty-three years later—that afternoon I visited with him—Dr. Louis Greenberg was still hunting the answers on arteriosclerosis. (Dr. Rinehart had died since their earlier work.)

As a pathologist at a great medical school, Dr. Louis Greenberg could speak with authority about arterial changes. "The monkeys were given the B_6-deficient diet when they were about one year old," he said. "They were fed this diet for a year to a year and a half. Some of the monkeys were preserved for about eight years. From time to time we would have to give them some B_6, else they would have died. It was our opinion that the longer the monkeys were on a B_6-deficient diet, the more nearly their arteriosclerosis resembled arteriosclerosis in the human."

Monkeys ordinarily live twenty to twenty-five years.

Critically analyzing the arteriosclerosis they found, Dr. Louis Greenberg said, "The monkey arteries showed a thickening of the intima [inner lining of the arteries], whereas control monkeys did not have this thickening. The lipid [fatty] deposition is different in human atherosclerosis as compared with experimental arteriosclerosis in the monkey."

It was the opinion of Dr. Greenberg, speaking as a pathologist, that persons who die of heart attacks have arteriosclerosis as the gross causative factor and high blood fats as an associated complicating factor. The Rinehart–Greenberg work with monkey arteriosclerosis was repeated by Drs. C. W. Mushett and Gladys Emerson, working in the Merck Company laboratories in the United States.[46] Dr. Greenberg also informed me that the same results were also produced by Kozo Yamada at Nagoya University School of Medicine, Nagoya, Japan.

In the early Rinehart–Greenberg work with rhesus monkeys, the test animals continued to eat well and gain weight for two to three weeks after pyridoxine was removed from the diet; after that point the food consumption fell off and the monkeys lost weight. Besides these changes and lessened vigor there was little change in appearance until five to six months after withdrawal of B_6. Then they became unkempt, sluggish, and hyperirritable when disturbed.

In this paper Rinehart and Greenberg reported pathologic examinations on five of the monkeys that had been on B_6-deficient diets for periods from five and a half to sixteen months. Although significant lesions were seen in the livers of two monkeys, the arterial lesions were "the most constant and prominent abnormality encountered." All five animals had sclerotic arterial lesions. The animals on the B_6-deficient diet for the longest periods, thirteen and sixteen months respectively, had the most widespread and advanced arteriosclerotic lesions. In addition to the coronary arteries, lesions were also prominent in the arteries of the kidney, pancreas, and elsewhere, including the arteries of the testicle in one animal. The scientists were greatly surprised to find advanced "arteriosclerosis" in the blood vessels of an immature testis. Plaques and patterns of distribution were among the features that paralleled arteriosclerosis in man. There seemed to be a change in the connective tissue substance of the intima. This and the fact that there was a blisterlike separation of tissues in some instances possibly were related to defective protein metabolism as a result of pyridoxine deficiency.

"There seems no question that the arterial lesions are related to pyridoxine deficiency," they concluded. "The experimental lesions . . . have a close resemblance to arteriosclerosis as it occurs in man." Because prolonged cholesterol feeding, by other researchers, had failed to produce such lesions in monkeys, there seemed to be a strong argument that the lesions occurred first and the cholesterol was deposited there afterward. Concluding, Rinehart and Greenberg wrote, "It is noteworthy that pyridoxine deficiency is in essence a chronic deficiency, relatively slow in evolution and without distinctive external manifestations. Such a deficiency state would be one particularly difficult of clinical recognition."[47]

Delving deeper into the biochemical mystery surrounding arteriosclerosis, other investigators have produced superbly refined data that fit into the Rinehart–Greenberg work and explain the mechanics of the lesions caused by B_6-deficient diet. British pathologist J. B. Gibson and associates, writing in the British Medical Association's *Journal of Clinical Pathology*, have reported on cases of mentally retarded children who had striking vascular lesions related to homocystinuria. Homocystine, the oxidized, disulfide form of homocysteine, is considered an abnormal metabolite of the essential sulphur-containing amino acid methionine, much as xanthurenic acid is an abnormal metabolite of tryptophan. In normal metabolism, methionine is broken down through homocysteine and cystathionine to cysteine and cystine. But homocystine had not been found in the normal metabolic pathway; thus, it is not normal to find it in urine.[48] When there is homocystinuria, or homocystine in the urine, something has gone wrong somewhere along the line. Some of the methionine has not been properly metabolized.

In 1969 pathologist Kilmer S. McCully, of the Harvest Medical School and the Massachusetts General Hospital, moved closer to the solution of the mystery when he proposed that an elevated homocysteine concentration, produced by B_6 deficiency, could explain the initial vascular damage in the monkeys Rinehart and Greenberg had tested. Since pyridoxine is a co-factor for cystathionine synthetase and for cystathionase, McCully saw the possibility that "pyridoxine deficiency produced elevated homocysteine concentration in the animals, leading to arterial damage and arteriosclerosis." McCully had found arterial lesions in a child with abnormal metabolism, and he saw a connection between that case and the Rinehart–Greenberg experiments. He attributed the lesions in the child and the ones found in other patients with a similar disorder to "the metabolic effects of increased concentrations of homocysteine, homocystine, or a derivative of homocysteine."[49]

An intensive researcher, McCully the next year reported: "The homocysteine effect on cellular proteoglycan synthesis is considered to be a key factor in the initiation of arteriosclerotic lesions because several lines of evidence from experimental and pathologic literature show that changes in sulfate esterified proteoglycans are an essential feature of the evolution of the arteriosclerotic process." McCully had studied cells cultured from the skin of individuals with cystathionine synthetase deficiency, and he produced the same results by adding homocysteine to the culture medium of normal cells. He was to conclude from these data that elevated concentrations of homocysteine will produce "pathologic changes in arteries and other connective tissues." On the basis of his interpretation of the laboratory results, he suggested restricting dietary methionine or administering choline and pyridoxine or possibly other measures, in order to prevent the arteriosclerotic lesions by reducing the concentrations of homocysteine in vascular cells.[50]

McCully and his associate, Bruce D. Ragsdale, later in 1970 proved that homocysteinemia, or homocysteine in the blood, rapidly produced arteriosclerotic plaques in laboratory rabbits, backing up McCully's previous work as well as that of Rinehart and Greenberg. Pointing out that the rabbit chow had a relatively high methionine content compared to the vegetarian diet consumed by wild rabbits, McCully and Ragsdale explained that animal proteins are more abundant in methionine than plant proteins. Many experimental atherogenic diets are high in methionine as well as cholesterol and other lipids. When cholesterol was added to the rabbits' diet, following the formation of lesions because of the homocysteine, then lipid deposits resulted in the aortic lesions. This suggested that cholesterol deposits were secondary and followed the primary vascular changes of homocysteinemia that damaged the elastic tissue.[51] There is, furthermore, the possibility—as yet unproved—that B_6 is involved, probably indirectly, in fat metabolism.[52]

The vital importance of B_6 is obvious. As Dr. Esmond E. Snell has stated, every amino acid that has been studied needs B_6 to complete its metabolism in the human body. This includes the amino acid methionine. If there is insufficient B_6 but a large intake of methionine in the diet, homocysteinemia is probable. A companion of homocysteinemia is the vascular lesion that we associate with arteriosclerosis, the dread forerunner of heart disease. In addition to dietary measures, it is clearly necessary that one have a sufficient daily supply of B_6 to help break down methionine as well as the other amino acids. But when arteriosclerosis is advanced, sufficient B_6 may not be enough. Once the lesions are far advanced, cholesterol probably will continue to collect. This would explain why B_6 hasn't been found to prevent heart attacks in older patients. They obviously will require B_6 and special dietary supervision that includes restriction of both methionine and cholesterol.

It seems apparent that enough evidence has been established in the laboratory and the clinic conclusively to associate vitamin B_6 deficiency with arteriosclerosis and the heart attack. Signs and symptoms in the hands and fingers of heart-attack victims in my clinic were responsive to pyridoxine. The methionine-B_6 relationship, also, might explain why epidemiologists have found less heart disease and less arteriosclerosis in countries where dietary animal protein is in better balance with vegetable protein—and where there is a greater intake of vitamin B_6.

PARKINSON'S DISEASE

In 1817 Dr. James Parkinson described a disease of the central nervous system that was characterized by rhythmic tremors of the resting muscles, usually in the legs and the hands. "Parkinson's disease" is found in persons around fifty to sixty years of age, and it may progress to the point where the patient has continuously shaking hands, arms, and legs, has to be confined to a chair, and has to be turned in bed with assistance. It is truly an agonizing disease.

Through studies of Parkinson's disease, vitamin B$_6$ has again become intimately associated with the physiology and metabolism of the brain. In a degradation of tyrosine, one of the amino acids, biochemists proved that the basal ganglia of the brain of patients with Parkinson's disease did not maintain a sufficient amount of dopamine and that large doses of L-dopa (levodopa) would restore dopamine to the basal ganglia to relieve the condition. It was soon learned, however, that doses of 10 to 25 milligrams of pyridoxine would interact with L-dopa and dopamine in these patients and render the L-dopa treatment ineffective. Some pharmaceutical houses even recommended B$_6$-deficient diets in an effort to enhance the effect of L-dopa.

However, Dr. Melvin Van Woert subsequently pointed out in the *Journal of the American Medical Association* that, for a number of reasons, it would be unwise to use a diet deficient in B$_6$. "Although a low pyridoxine diet might be expected to increase the proportion of levodopa reaching the brain," stated Van Woert, "other factors suggest that the use of this diet could be an unwise or even dangerous procedure." Examining the specific biochemical reactions involved, Van Woert reasoned that "the ingestion of large amounts of levodopa may produce a relative or absolute pyridoxine deficiency." Levodopa, he further pointed out, inhibits pyridoxal kinase, the enzyme that converts pyridoxal to its active coenzyme, pyridoxal 5' phosphate.

"With a regular diet," Van Woert wrote, "the obvious clinical signs of severe pyridoxine deficiency, e.g. convulsions, peripheral neuropathy, dermatitis, have not developed in patients treated with levodopa. However, long-term administration of levodopa in conjunction with a low pyridoxine diet might conceivably produce a serious vitamin-deficiency state. In my opinion, the undemonstrated clinical benefit and questionable rationale for combining a low pyridoxine diet with levodopa does not warrant the widespread use of this potentially dangerous mode of therapy. A limited controlled investigation to evaluate this treatment during which the patient is protected by sophisticated monitoring of his condition is justified, and should have preceded the general distribution of the low pyridoxine diet."[53] A subsequent experiment with mice by other investigators supported the contention that "pyridoxine is not contra-indicated in patients receiving a combination of levodopa and peripheral decarboxylase inhibitors, but rather may result in further enhancement of therapeutic effect."[54]

What is of utmost importance here is that levodopa information inserts, included by the drug companies, carry the legend required by the Food and Drug Administration that its "long-term safety and efficacy has not been established." On the other hand, B_6's long-term safety and efficacy and, in fact, its vital role have all been established. In my own experience I have given from 50 to 100 milligrams of pyridoxine to patients who had Parkinson's disease, and I was unable to detect any way in which it may have made the patients any worse; nor, having given pyridoxine to hundreds of elderly persons with various forms of weakness and tremors, was I ever to see that pyridoxine triggered or precipitated Parkinson's disease.

It is my opinion that, since L-dopa will have to be given under the guidance of a physician, he be allowed to determine the amount of vitamin B_6 the patient should receive. It seems only logical, however, that the vitamin B_6 contained in a well-balanced diet should not be sacrificed in order to use L-dopa. What is of great significance to us here is that in Parkinson's disease another amino acid, tyrosine, high in the brain and involved in brain metabolism, was found to be associated intimately with B_6.

DENTAL CARIES

There is some evidence that pyridoxine is a factor in the prevention of tooth decay. Citing clinical studies that indicate pyridoxine lozenges reduced caries in school children as much as 50 percent, Robert W. Hillman of the Downstate Medical Center in Brooklyn has suggested a number of ways in which B_6 may help prevent tooth decay. Other data indicate that B_6 "may be among the protective elements lost in the sugar refining process." Cuban children who chew sugar cane had fewer caries and higher blood concentrations of B$_6$ than did a peer group in New York City, reported two studies cited by Hillman.[55] Rinehart and Greenberg also clearly demonstrated that the young, developing monkeys on a B$_6$-deficient diet had devastating tooth decay, whereas control monkeys did not.[56] Long-range investigations are needed to determine if children given 10 milligrams of pyridoxine daily, along with adequate minerals, can be prevented from having tooth decay.

KIDNEY STONES

Dr. Stanley N. Gershoff, of the department of nutrition at the Harvard School of Public Health, has reported laboratory studies that implicate both B$_6$ and magnesium deficiencies in renal, or kidney, stones. He demonstrated that high levels of dietary magnesium protect against renal oxalate deposits in B$_6$-deficient rats; it did not, however, decrease the level of oxalate in the urine that the deficiency had caused. Xanthurenic acid also was "significantly increased when vitamin B$_6$-deficient rats are fed diets low in magnesium." When there is a B$_6$ deficiency there is also a "marked decrease" in urinary citrate. This can be prevented by ingestion of high magnesium levels. Citric acid may help dissolve calcium oxalate.

B$_6$ and magnesium seem to work in different ways to combat kidney stones. B$_6$ has an effect on oxalate metabolism, while magnesium probably alters the solvent characteristics of urine.

In previous work Gershoff had found an increase in oxalate excretion when the tryptophan load test was given to human subjects. The amino acid tryptophan is a precursor of oxalate in rats; its faulty metabolism is a likely early step in the forming of stones.

In other human studies Gershoff and associates reported that even when the subjects were apparently receiving sufficient B$_6$ from their diets and were not excreting oxalate excessively, B$_6$ supplementation nonetheless caused a decrease in urinary oxalate. This led the scientists to this interesting conclusion: "It would appear that for many, it not all, individuals, the dietary level of vitamin B_6 needed to ensure minimal oxalate excretion is greater than the amount needed to protect against most other known manifestations of vitamin B_6 deficiency."[57]

SUMMARY

One must understand that it is most difficult for a clinician to evaluate patients by fixed criteria or standards. No two hands are exactly alike. No two shoulders are exactly similar. One shoulder may be painful, the other not painful. Because of these differences I have found my most useful variable, over and over, to be the time factor during which the patient responded to B_6 therapy. Experience established this time factor at from three to six weeks. If a patient could not grasp his razor with enough strength to shave himself for three months, yet after three weeks of B_6 therapy he could clutch a hoe and work in his garden, it seemed evident that B_6 could be credited with the change. This occurred over and over.

I sometimes found it necessary to combine other medication with B_6 for optimum improvement of symptoms, particularly in the shoulders. It has been proved that rheumatism is responsive to the adrenocorticotropic hormone (ACTH) and other steroids, such as estrogen. As we have now seen in this book, vitamin B_6 is important in the clinical relief of rheumatism in the shoulders, arms, and hands. Because of the biochemical relationship of B_6 to estrogen, as proved in the laboratory, there must be a general relationship in the clinic between B_6 and the steroid hormones, and this may well include ACTH. Viewing cases such as that of a man with very painful and stiffened shoulders, I acquired the opinion that in some cases the pain and stiffness responded better to a few small doses of both ACTH and pyridoxine than to ACTH alone or B_6 alone. Regardless of use of ACTH, patients with the shoulder-hand syndrome were maintained on pyridoxine (50 to 100 milligrams daily and indefinitely).

I hesitate even to mention ACTH in this discussion, because critics will maintain that no standard of evaluation could be established regarding the use of B_6. But I must emphasize that many patients had the complete hand symptomatology, as well as shoulders so painful that they couldn't sleep or rest on them at night; yet when their hand symptoms improved, so did their shoulder symptoms—simultaneously and in the same time interval of from three to six weeks, with B₆ the only therapy.

Some critics will maintain that a certain percentage of the patients with carpal tunnel syndrome will improve, regardless of treatment. To some degree this may be granted. However, if those patients are followed up long enough, they will be found still to have diffuse edema in the hands, as well as a continuation of paresthesia from time to time. In such cases, when pyridoxine was given, both edema and paresthesia subsided—invariably within three to six weeks. This occurred despite the fact, as reported by George S. Phalen, an authority, that patients with carpal tunnel syndrome have a symptomatology that sometimes has existed for years. I personally have had patients who stated they had suffered from all these symptoms for years. A similar pattern has developed in the treatment of other conditions that have responded to B₆.

In this book I have described a large number of cases that attest to the medicinal values of B₆. In this chapter, especially, supporting evidence from the laboratory has been presented to back up my clinical findings. However, I wish to point out that results found in animal research in the laboratory are sometimes a thing apart from results obtained with human patients. I have researched the medical literature many times on a number of subjects and I have learned that one can prove almost anything with at least three papers on a given subject. A good example of this is the role of fat in the diet. By selecting articles from the literature, one can prove it either way, that fat is good for one or that fat is bad for one.

But when one has objective evidence of clinical improvement of signs and symptoms in the human, it transcends anything seen anywhere else. It is proof positive. And when laboratory and clinical data form a dovetail, there can be no doubt.

The Future:
A Projection for B₆ | 12

The final picture of B_6's role remains incomplete, as scientists continue to put the pieces together, but the puzzle is moving closer to solution each year because, in the words of Paul György, "At present we are facing an almost explosive interest in the metabolic role of vitamin B_6 in man."[1]

From what we already know, B_6's role in metabolism is at least as complicated as the workings of a fifty-cylinder automobile. In order for that automobile to operate as it should, its engine must be hitting on all fifty cylinders. If it is not, it is not in proper working order. The same is true for the human body and the more than fifty enzymatic reactions related to B_6. If there is inadequate B_6 in order for those reactions to occur, then the body is not in proper working order. It is in ill health, and the severity of the disorder depends on the degree of the deficiency.

I do not wish to give the impression that vitamin B_6 is the only nutrient necessary for prevention of disease. All vitamins and minerals are important. A delicate balance of the other vitamins and minerals that act and interact with B_6 is also necessary in order for each nutrient to function properly and to be utilized by the body. Although there clearly is a B_6-deficiency disease, this does not mean that B_6 is necessarily the only nutrient lacking in many patients. They very likely may be deficient in other vitamins and

205

minerals as well. This has been shown to be especially true of magnesium. For this reason, it is usually necessary to improve a patient's general diet, along with B_6 supplementation. Establishment of the optimum amount of nature's nutrients for human health is a fascinating challenge that makes the study of food so important and interesting.

What is most significant is that vitamin B_6 is the protein vitamin, without which protein cannot be utilized properly, in a land where more protein is eaten than virtually any other nation on earth. And, as R. R. Brown has suggested, "Although this vitamin is widely distributed in a variety of foods, its content in foods eaten by a weight conscious population may be rather marginal." As Brown has also explained, even adequate intake may not be sufficient. There are factors that may make for a tissue deficiency: impaired delivery of the vitamin or excessive loss of the vitamin through excretion or through inactivation with chemicals and drugs.[2] Enzymatic defects also may be involved.[3]

Henry Borsook of the California Institute of Technology, reviewing the amounts of B_6 in diets, has reported the *lowest* loss of B_6 in the cooking of meat as 18 percent but with *most figures* between 20 and 25 percent, with some as high as *70 percent*. In vegetables, 20 to 30 percent is destroyed; canned foods lose accordingly. Only frozen processing seems to preserve the B_6. In processing wheat flour, 80 to 90 percent of the B_6 is taken out with the bran, and the baking costs 3.5 to 17.5 percent of the B_6. He quoted surveys that indicate a large proportion of American adults is not getting 1.5 milligrams daily—too low—and one Cincinnati hospital provided only 1.0 to 1.5 milligrams in the diet.[4]

We have seen that many, many Americans have an increased need for vitamin B_6. They, and probably many others, will need more vitamin B_6. But one hesitates to comment as to where and how pyridoxine should be added as a food supplement until, first, a concept of deficiency has been either accepted or rejected. Several questions logically arise. What is B_6 deficiency? What is B_6 dependency? What is an increased need for B_6? Some scientists, supported by sound reasons, may maintain that some individuals need more B_6 than do others and that the signs and symptoms I have described do not represent deficiency but rather represent an

increased need for the vitamin in that particular person
foregoing pages of this book I have honored that concept
to prevent the formation of some sort of bias before the evi...
could be presented. If my patients have inborn errors of metabolism and an unusually high requirement for pyridoxine, then
this is not vitamin B_6 deficiency. It seems clear to me, however,
that many, certainly, of my patients have had B_6 deficiency. The
reduction of edema and all the symptomatology that is associated
in so many, many patients leads me to believe that they had a
deficiency condition rather than some inborn abnormality. I cannot
accept that this symptomatology is confined to northeast Texas.
Patients with acroparesthesia and rheumatism responsive to B_6
could be found and treated daily in every large clinic in the
civilized world. *I have seen enough husbands and wives who ate
from the same table and who suffered from the same symptomatology to conclude positively that vitamin B_6 deficiency is the most
prevalent deficiency disease in the United States today.* On the
basis of my observations of these couples alone one would be
compelled to discount that it was strictly an enzymatic defect
attributable to heredity. In other words, we have no alternative
but to accept the concept that massive B_6 deficiency exists, and
this widespread deficiency must be dealt with just as forcefully as
were beriberi, pellagra, and scurvy.

The ideal way to get sound nutrition, if one is not starting out
too far behind, is through a proper diet, high in foods that have
naturally existing B_6. But when a person is deficient, and this
deficiency is long-standing, how is one to regain all the years of lost
ground without supplementing his proper diet with B_6 tablets? I
have never sold a single B_6 tablet in my life, nor do I ever expect
to benefit financially from the use of B_6. But there is no getting
around the fact that millions of Americans need B_6 supplements.

How much B_6 should one take each day if one wants to take
supplements? Not knowing the exact amount that might be needed
for each individual, I would recommend that a more than adequate
amount be taken, which would be 50 milligrams daily for all those
not pregnant and 100 to 300 milligrams daily for those who are
pregnant, depending on the amount of edema and the signs of
acroparesthesia or carpal tunnel syndrome.

Any excess of pyridoxine is excreted in the urine within eight hours. When the dosage is divided, I recommend that 50 milligrams be taken after breakfast and 50 milligrams after the evening meal if, for example, one is taking 100 milligrams daily. Even more ideal would be 50 milligrams following each of the three meals, if one is taking a total of 150 milligrams daily.

After eleven years of investigations involving thousands of patients, each taking from 50 to 400 milligrams of pyridoxine hydrochloride daily, I have observed no serious side effects except in persons who had duodenal ulcers. These patients complained of more gastric or stomach disturbance. I discussed this with Dr. Louis Greenberg. The thought occurred to him, and it seems reasonable to me, that the hydrochloride radical of pyridoxine hydrochloride might have contributed to the gastric complaints of these patients with duodenal ulcers. Work needs to be done to determine if these patients will tolerate better the pyridoxal phosphate form of the vitamin.

As for very high dosages, I observed one fifty-one-year-old woman who for fifteen years had suffered with idiopathic edema; within a few hours she often would gain as much as fifteen pounds. At her request I gave her 1,000 milligrams of pyridoxine hydrochloride daily for thirteen days. Serum electrolyte studies were done near the beginning and at the close of the study. Serum electrolyte studies became more nearly normal by the end of the study, and her idiopathic edema, previously treated in some very reputable clinics, had been completely relieved.

Some very good writers have stated that a balance of B_2 and B_6 is needed, but I have not seen any appearance of riboflavin deficiency when I gave large doses of B_6. In my opinion, a quantitative balance of B_2 and B_6 is not necessary.

Furthermore, in light of these widespread deficiency conditions in this country, it is my opinion, as it is Paul György's, that the minimum daily requirements for B_6 should be changed from the present 2 to 2.5 milligrams daily to 25 milligrams a day. There also should be 100 milligrams of B_6 in every prenatal capsule and 50 milligrams in each supplementary vitamin tablet for therapeutic use. It is also my firm conviction, after eleven years of clinical studies with the vitamin, that the minimum daily requirements for all infants and children under twelve years of age should be set at 10 milligrams. When these concepts are accepted, in my opinion a lot of disease is going to disappear in the civilized world. The old idea of establishing as the minimum daily requirement that amount on which a *majority* of the people can *survive* must be abandoned. It leaves an insufficiency for a large minority, and this constitutes a dangerous gap. As biochemist Roger J. Williams has so carefully demonstrated, there are wide differences in the requirements of many individuals.

All women on birth-control pills should take 50 milligrams of pyridoxine daily. Every time a woman takes an antiovulatory pill she should also take a B$_6$ pill. In fact, B$_6$ and the Pill might well be combined by pharmaceutical houses into a single medication.

All pregnant women need even greater B$_6$ supplements at the beginning of pregnancy, at a time when they do not often know they are pregnant, which is a strong argument for routine supplementation of B$_6$ for all women of child-bearing age. Whatever the source, women need more B$_6$ when estrogen is increased, as in the Pill, or produced, as in pregnancy. As for men, there is a puzzling little fact of endocrinology that may indicate men, too, may routinely require more B$_6$ than we have previously believed. There is one half as much estradiol, a female hormone, in the urine of men as of women. There is as much female hormone in the testicle of a stallion as in any other known tissue. Its significance, especially in regard to B$_6$, is yet to be spelled out.

B$_6$ must become a routine supplementation for pregnant women in the prenatal clinics around the world. A minimum of 100 milligrams daily should be given every pregnant woman, without waiting to see if she has the complications of edema. If she develops edema her dosage should be increased to 400 milligrams a day, along with 1,000 milligrams of magnesium oxide daily as an adjunctive supplement.

Meanwhile, long-range investigations should be undertaken to determine the effects of magnesium and pyridoxine on insulin secretion during pregnancy. In fact, extensive and long-range studies on the relationship of B$_6$ and magnesium in the possible prevention of diabetes might be most rewarding.

It has long been established that maternal care must begin early in the prenatal period. With the increased knowledge that we now have of B_6, we approach this with a greater sense of urgency. Vitamins prevent birth defects. We have seen this over and over with animals. Professor Fred Hale, in work at the Texas A & M University Experiment Station, showed that hogs on a special deficiency diet produced litters in which the young had cleft palates and other birth defects. He proved that vitamin A was necessary in the diet of mammals to prevent birth defects. His work was the "first clear proof that a nutritional deficiency could produce congenital malformations in mammals."[5]

The same has been proved for B_6. B_6 deficiency has caused very severe birth defects in laboratory rats. The human animal is not exempt from the same laws of nature. Based on evidence I have seen in my own clinic, I am positive that edematous infants are being born of edematous mothers and that B_6 will relieve edema in both. Maternal and infant nutrition must be improved in this country, and B_6 must become one of the first defensive weapons in the prevention of birth defects.

B_6 should become a part of the infant's daily dietary, as soon as he is born. If the infant is on breast milk, the mother should be placed on B_6 supplements. The infant should receive 10 milligrams of B_6 daily during the first year of life to insure complete brain development and also because it cannot be determined yet which infant has a high requirement for the nutrient.

As of now, supplementing the American diet with B_6 may not be so easily done. Today we have a scarcity of B_6 supplements. Drug manufacturers do not commonly make it. Until 1968 vitamin B_6 was not recognized by the National Research Council in a recommended daily requirement. The recommended dose was very low. It ranged from 0.2 milligrams for babies to a high of 2.5 milligrams for a pregnant or lactating woman. Drug-house representatives have appeared in my office throughout the past decade in which I have done my clinical work with B_6 and I have never heard one mention using B_6 for anything except in the treatment of tuberculosis. At the time of this writing, only three U. S. companies manufacture B_6. Obviously we must have a more plentiful supply of B_6 supplements if we are to overcome the deficiency and prevent future deficiency conditions.

Unfortunately, it is probable that during the lifetime of every person living today, supplements will be necessary, for there are few, if any, Americans, certainly, who have received the optimum daily intake of B_6 from fetal life to the present. Supplementation is the only way left in which to overcome what is probably some degree of deficiency as a result of our having eaten food that is either overcooked, overprocessed, or to some extent depleted or devoid of B_6.

Not only must the American diet be improved in B_6 content; it also must provide for an increased intake of magnesium, one of the significant co-factors of B_6. Both agricultural and laboratory evidence supports this need. People must be trained in proper nutrition so that they will know the foods that are highest in magnesium, just as they must know which foods provide them sufficient vitamin B_6. Nuts and cereals are among the best suppliers of magnesium, followed in order by sea foods, meats, legumes, vegetables, and fruits. At the bottom of the lists of all foods, with respect to vitamins and minerals, are refined sugars and fats. While fats and refined sugars provide a giant portion of calories in this country, they are virtually devoid of magnesium. Furthermore, magnesium, like B_6 and other vitamins and minerals, is lost through refining of raw foods and by cooking. Dr. Henry A. Schroeder and associates, in studies at Dartmouth Medical School and Brattleboro Memorial Hospital, reported, "The refining of whole wheat to fine patent flour resulted in a loss of 80 per cent of the magnesium, as it did for the essential trace elements. . . . The polishing of rice may remove more than 80 per cent of the magnesium. The refinement of sugar removed nearly all of the magnesium in sugar cane or in raw sugar, with a consequent marked enrichment of molasses. Boiling vegetables in water removed more than half of the magnesium from celery, two-thirds from carrots and nearly three-quarters from parsnips." The researchers pointed out that "the enriched residues from the refined carbohydrates of wheat and sugar cane are fed to poultry and livestock, whereas human beings eat the depleted material."

Schroeder and his colleagues explained: "*From the viewpoint of the evolutionary dietary history of the human race, it is logical to believe that every major natural source of caloric energy carries with it the inorganic nutrients necessary for its metabolism. This statement holds for all animals; otherwise deficiencies would occur and species would either become extinct or would have to depend on more than one source of food for survival (i.e. a 'balanced' diet)."* But balanced diets are necessary for domestic and laboratory animals and for man, the researchers continue, because pastures are overcropped or otherwise depleted of trace elements, while at the same time foods are prepared from many sources and are processed in many ways. They state that they know of no wild animal on land or sea that requires a "balanced" diet.[6]

Although most doctors will, I believe, accept the evidence and findings in this book, many rheumatologists probably will remain skeptical of the medicinal effects of B₆. Many probably will not prescribe B₆ for the shoulder-hand syndrome because in a number of cases there has been and will be recurrence of shoulder and elbow pain. Yet to me the association seems too strong to ignore. When the carpal tunnel syndrome is full-blown, the patient also has shoulder and elbow pains; such a frequent association is almost assuredly related. Of all physicians, rheumatologists are most likely to be agnostic toward B₆. When one discusses the carpal tunnel syndrome, for example, one is likely to get this response from them: "Well, a certain percent of carpal tunnel syndrome patients get better even if you don't do anything." This may be true, but it does not take into account cases like that of our seamstress N. H. in Chapter 9. This woman had been on government subsidies, unable to work for six months. Yet within three weeks she—like many others—was virtually cured. The time factor alone was powerful documentation for B₆ in the field of rheumatology.

Furthermore, in the cases in which the patient reputedly got better spontaneously, the patients invariably continued to suffer from paresthesia, and they still had diffuse edema—even after they "got better." But when treated with B₆ they got better *and* found relief from paresthesia and edema. Does not this difference in clinical behavior argue B₆'s case as forcibly as it can be done?

I don't think it is unethical to meet counterpoints head on. Inevitably, critics may be expected to charge that results with pyridoxine are not immediate and complete; that is to say, it does not

---

* Italics added.

give 100 percent results. But I do not hold that we must have results as dramatic as those gained in the cure of beriberi, night blindness, and pellagra. I do not claim 100 percent. In some cases, the patient has had his disorder for such a length of time that one cannot always expect immediate positive results. But the overwhelming general results are positive, as shown in the earlier chapters of this book, and I personally am just as interested in improvement of 20 percent of the patients with shoulder symptoms as supporters of vitamin B_1 are interested in relieving 100 percent of their patients with beriberi. I think most doctors are interested in getting the best results they can get, even if that best is only 10 to 20 percent of the patients or symptoms. Twenty percent is better than zero. What is of overwhelming importance is that, based on eleven years of clinical experience with thousands of patients, virtually 100 percent of the patients with acroparesthesia can be relieved with pyridoxine. When the recovery rate is that high, there is no doubt whatsoever as to the effectiveness of B_6.

But in some cases, in some patients, 15 or 20 percent effect is significant. It may be the best a doctor can do. For this reason, even in those patients who do not seem to enjoy a full recovery from the symptoms for which pyridoxine is usually helpful, the vitamin is advisable as therapy for partial results. There is no getting around the fact that, when nothing else has done the job, a 20 percent effectiveness is important. It is important, most of all, to those patients who make up that 20 percent.

There will be a temptation by some critics, I am sure, to insist that more laboratory evidence should have accompanied these studies in northeast Texas. Other critics will say that much of the subjective symptomatology improves, disappears, and then recurs in a certain number of persons. I am willing to accept both criticisms. Yet no criticism can override the facts presented in photographic evidence showing before-and-after treatment with pyridoxine. Numerous patients also demonstrate in motion pictures how pyridoxine objectively improved their conditions. These are unalterable objective documentation of the physiological response. Always, that time factor of three to six weeks was important in documenting response to pyridoxine.

As for double-blind studies, I am not adverse at all to having my clinical findings carefully checked by skilled technicians and by other doctors. But the nature of my practice, in a small town in northeast Texas, is not such that it is a simple matter to find new patients that one might use in such a study. Over the years those patients who exhibited these signs and symptoms we have discussed were treated with B_6. Therefore, in order to conduct double-blind studies I would have to acquire new patients with similar symptomatology—patients who had not yet received pyridoxine. It would be almost impossible for me to do such a thing in my general practice in Mt. Pleasant, Texas, a town of 14,000 where drugstores commonly sell 100,000 B_6 tablets a month. It would be hard to find a patient who has not taken B_6. And in some patients the problem is imposing. For instance, how can a double-blind study be done on patients with bowel obstruction, with and without diabetes? The patients are all different, in different respects. But I hope that doctors elsewhere will check this work with double-blind studies of their own.

The most important thing to any physician is that his patients be given the best, most up-to-date medical attention for his symptoms. When a substance or medication works for a specific disorder, and it is known that it works, then it should be used, whether there has been a double-blind study or not. This principle was recognized in a 1972 editorial by the publisher of *Medical Tribune and Medical News*, Arthur M. Sackler, M.D., in which he pointed out that finally, after forty years of use, gold salts had been proved, by a double-blind test, to be helpful in treating rheumatoid arthritis. Dr. Sackler wrote:

> The painful fact remains that thousands of victims of rheumatoid arthritis denied gold salt therapy may have suffered cartilage damage, bone erosion, restricted mobility, and pain, which could have been either arrested or deferred in time, while awaiting a "ritual" double-blind clarification of what was apparently clinically clear to observant rheumatologists. Granted the limitations of the benefits of gold salt therapy, patients can have small comfort either in hindsight or in the fact that it took 40 years for the double-blind study to confirm the clarity of vision and therapeutic insight of good clinicians.

I hope I will not be charged with being overly partisan when I suggest that this logic is even more pertinent to the clinical use of B$_6$. If for no other reason, B$_6$ affects a greater number of persons than does gold-salt therapy. Although the various disorders may be related, or at least associated in a number of patients, B$_6$ may—and should—be taken by patients ranging from the young pregnant to the elderly. Those fifty enzymatic reactions it aids are important to all of us.

There is a large gap between the clinic and the laboratory in techniques. The laboratory can demand precision in techniques and results in dealing with experimental animals. But in the clinic this is not so, and cannot be so, because one is dealing with human beings. Many diagnoses must necessarily be educated guesses because even diagnostic tests are not always definitive; moreover, a doctor cannot be certain, in all diseases, as to which test to give a patient. In the clinic the human factor is always present. Observation and judgment are the great factors in dealing with human patients. And in making a diagnosis and prescribing treatment, a physician's powers of observation are likely to be his most effective tool for detecting and relieving disease.

The significance of clinical observation was driven home forcibly to me one day in the nineteen sixties by Dr. Jan Bonsma of the University of Praetoria, South Africa. Dr. Bonsma was teaching that year at Texas A & M University, having taken a sabbatical from his South African post. He was an authority on animal husbandry. He had been brought to the United States because of his work in cattle production. As mentioned previously, Dr. Bonsma had recognized certain features of cows that were dependent on their hormonal development; these features, he had discovered, were also related to the fertility of the animals. That day as I accompanied him about a large South Texas ranch I received an indelible impression of his sharply discriminating powers of observation. As the animals trotted past him he separated them, after visually examining them, into two groups, one on either side of the nearby highway. Yet in this seemingly casual way he managed to divide, with a great degree of success, the animals that proved to have a poor calving record from those on the other side of the highway that had a high fertility, better calf-producing record. How did he do it? He had a trained eye and he knew what he was looking for.

That day, as we stood in the cow pasture and quietly talked, he told me, "*It is the observation of the slight deviation from the normal that makes a good doctor. If one observes more thoroughly than the other, then he is the better doctor.*"

It was the dermatitis of a rat's ear that first guided Paul György toward the eventual discovery of vitamin B_6, and it was his observation that the experimental rats were not growing properly that assisted materially in the discovery of riboflavin. It was the same slight deviation from normal in my patients' hands and fingers, before treatment, compared with their appearance after treatment with pyridoxine, that caused me to conclude that I was seeing an increased need for B_6 in hundreds of persons.

Our well-known historical deficiency diseases were much easier defined. Beriberi was as big as the Far East and was readily recognized. Scurvy, as large as the Seven Seas on which it occurred, was easily recognized by any old sailor on the long voyages. Xerophthalmia of vitamin A deficiency was as obvious as the blindness it caused, and rickets, the vitamin D deficiency, was as prominent as the bowed legs of children who were deficient in vitamin D. Although in this book we have described more pathology, and more patients, than have been described for a deficiency disorder since Goldberger studied pellagra, the signs and symptoms of what appears to be vitamin B_6 deficiency have been perceived and described with difficulty. But if this B_6 deficiency had been as obvious as Pike's Peak, it would have been discovered long ago. Yet it is probably one of the most rampant deficiency disorders facing this country today. Most deficiency diseases by now have been brought under control—pellagra, scurvy, rickets, etc. I haven't seen five cases of real pernicious anemia—caused by vitamin B_{12} deficiency —since I have been practicing medicine. But in eleven years I have treated hundreds of severe, and thousands of milder, cases of B_6 deficiency.

Non-scientists must realize that studies of the vitamins have been tedious and time-consuming. Conclusions have been arrived at with great difficulty. Paul György, as we have seen, worked twelve years before he presented his first paper on biotin. This is as it should be, for the true scientist is interested, most of all, in what is the truth and what it will mean to the ones who follow him. In this spirit, as we have prepared the material for this book we have looked for the *proved* facts that can be depended on as a firm basis for future laboratory investigations. The overstatement does not belong in science. Pursuit of the untenable is not a part of science. And if there is one line in this book that is an overstatement or is untenable, we, the authors, are not aware of it.

I have learned much from my association with some of the great scientists who have worked with B_6 in the laboratory and in the universities. And I have learned more than the facts they contributed. They have given of themselves, too, of their personalities, and I have been blessed by my association with them.

Of these, none has been more generous than Paul György. It was he who introduced me, by letter, to Dr. Roger J. Williams, another pioneer scientist in the story of the B-complex vitamins. Dr. Williams, in turn, invited me to present my motion pictures and audio-tape recordings of patients to him and his colleagues at the Clayton Foundation Biochemical Institute at the University of Texas in Austin.

The day I went to Austin became a memorable one to me for both personal and professional reasons. Some time before my younger daughter, Joan, had returned home to await the birth of her first child. Another doctor was to deliver the baby, but she wanted to have Daddy near. On the day I was to go to Austin I knew she would give birth soon. I was in a dilemma. But Joan knew how much it meant to me to present my findings to the biochemists at the University of Texas. She urged me to go.

As I drove to Austin early that morning, unaware of what was going on at home, Joan went into labor. She entered the hospital in Mt. Pleasant. Hours later, while I showed my motion pictures to Dr. Williams and his colleagues in a personal effort to bridge the gap between laboratory and clinic, my daughter gave birth to my first grandson. The date, May 26, 1971, was etched indelibly in my mind. It was nine years to the day since I had injected pyridoxine into the arm of a pregnant woman in an attempt to control edema.

Roger Williams had spent the major portion of his life in the study of nutrition, and, as I was to learn that day, he had seen, in his earlier years, some of the ravaging results of B-vitamin deficiency. I asked him where he had been born. "India," he said. He was the son of a missionary. As a child he had seen beriberi at first hand. In the nineteen thirties his brother, Dr. Robert R. Williams, separated the first ounce of pure thiamine (vitamin B_1), the substance that would cure the terrible, deadly beriberi of India and the Far East. The role of nutrition in individual and national health was nothing new to Roger Williams.

Paul György has not only brought me into contact with great scientists; he also has personally inspired me over and over. He visited me at my Texas home in 1970 and again in 1971, with Mrs. György accompanying him on the second trip. Paul is a scientist of the highest order, a man with a precision of mind that allows no unproved statement to masquerade as truth. One would expect this of a scientist who labored twelve years before finally publishing a paper on a particular subject of research, as he did on biotin.

During those visits to Texas, when I began "thinking out loud," he would become critical of my musings and speculations.

"If you haven't proven it, don't say it—keep it to yourself," he would admonish, in a firm but not harsh tone in his exotic Hungarian accent.

This I could understand and appreciate. He is a man who stimulates a person to do better work. But Paul didn't understand the musings of a country doctor. My father went to a medical meeting in East Texas many years ago and heard somebody say there were three characteristics of a country doctor: unpressed pants, a peculiar case to relate, and horse manure on his shoes. I will confess to having at least one of those characteristics. I have a peculiar case to relate.

A woman near the age of menopause from West Texas, hundreds of miles away, was visiting relatives in East Texas. She had extensive edema in her face, hands, feet, and ankles. She had been taking diuretics and four grains of thyroid extract daily. I gave her 50 milligrams of B_6 daily and told her to reduce the thyroid extract to one grain daily and to discontinue the diuretics. She went home to West Texas. Three months later she returned to East Texas, and when she arrived at the front door her relative didn't recognize her at first. She had lost so much edema in her face and her face was so wrinkled, consequently, that she seemed to be another person.

I am reporting this not as a conclusion but as a clue for future researchers, for as Paul György would caution this is a projection for the future. Other investigators have said myxedema is associated with the carpal tunnel syndrome. Possibly, as in this "peculiar case," B6 in some way affects or improves thyroid function or utilization of thyroxin. It has been shown that more pyridoxine is needed for the increased utilization of estrogen, and there is reason to believe that pyridoxine is important in the utilization of other hormones. One of our future concerns must be with determining the role of B6 in its support of the endocrine glands themselves and in the utilization of the hormones they produce.

Only time will tell the full story of damage that vitamin B6 deficiency has caused. But the American people are now suffering from B6 deficiency, and the deficiency seems very prevalent in this country. Apparently there are two major reasons for this situation: consumption of foods containing insufficient natural supplies of B6 and destruction of naturally occurring B6 in foods by processing and overcooking. For instance, lean beef has two to three times as much B6 as vegetables, but the cooking of meats destroys much of the B6, while the amino acids are fairly stable to heat. Presumably, before cooking, the protein in the meat was accompanied by enough B6 to insure the process of metabolism. But the process of cooking lowers the B6 consumed—while increasing the need for it. The greatest fault of frying may be, after all, not so much the fats used as the *heat*.

Facing a vicious set of circumstances such as these, the human being would have no way to take in, through food, a high enough level of B6 each day. No person is likely to take in more than 5 milligrams of B6 daily from food, because of its relative rarity. It may be possible that thousands and millions of years earlier man did not face this B6 destruction from cooking, for there was a time when man ate his meat raw, or at least very rare. There is even a vast difference today from the nutritional environment of the last century, or even that of the earlier years of this century. Both of my grandfathers—Grandpa Speer on my mother's side, Grandfather Ellis on my father's—lived to be near ninety years old; neither one ever took a vitamin supplement. Something besides heredity seemed to be at work. But today much is complicated by the fact that too many of us eat food that has little or no B_6, a dietary conditioning and the result of overprocessing and overcooking of food that has left millions of sick Americans. In fact, numbers of my patients, themselves suffering from chronic B_6 deficiency, were cooks in schools, hotels, restaurants, and hospitals. Much of the B_6 they so desperately needed they had destroyed themselves!

In the clinic, the adoption of one simple test could lead to early detection of thousands and thousands—perhaps millions—of early cases of B_6 deficiency. I am referring to the Quick Early Warning (QEW) finger flexion test I have described. The QEW test is established; it can be used around the world and it can determine, in a matter of seconds, if a patient is deficient in B_6 at the clinical level. This simple test, consisting of flexing fingertips to the metacarpophalangeal crease of the hand, can be given by a medical technician or assistant after a few minutes of instruction from the physician. As clinical evidence of B_6 deficiency, it is quick, reliable, and graphic, and it can be administered with no loss of time. The QEW test is much more simple than the breast-lump check or the Pap smear for, respectively, breast cancer and cervix cancer. It should be given routinely in any medical checkup. A patient could be readily trained to administer it to himself, and any reader of this book should be equipped to do so by now.

The future of B_6 in the U. S. hospitals and clinics will depend on better methods of assay, which is now difficult to perform and expensive to produce. Few hospitals routinely check to see if the patients have vitamin deficiencies of any sort; neither is the serum magnesium routinely checked in this country's hospitals. Medical students need to be taught more about nutrition. The entire food industry needs a new point of view relative to nutrition.

On the basis of present clinical knowledge, more intensified research is needed on vitamin B_6. This need breaks down into several areas of investigation, including the following.

1. While B_6 must become the routine medication for rheumatism, the type most frequently encountered in the civilized world,

research is needed to discover precisely how the vitamin works to relieve symptoms and signs.

2. Pyridoxine should be used in lieu of diuretics in many cases, becoming an accepted therapeutic agent in controlling edema, and *an unending search must be made to determine the process whereby B₆ relieves edema.*

3. Investigations are needed in the effects of pyridoxine hydrochloride in treating patients who also have duodenal ulcers. I am convinced that these patients need additional antacid therapy if they take pyridoxine hydrochloride.

4. A detailed and exhaustive study is necessary of the two cofactors, pyridoxine and magnesium, in treating of diabetes, epilepsy, heart disease, and eclampsia.

5. The relationship of B₆ deficiency with diabetes and arteriosclerosis should be a long-range study goal. B₆ deficiency in animals and fowl definitely causes arterial disease. I have demonstrated clinical response to B₆ in numbers of diabetic patients as well as those suffering from heart disease. Diabetes, heart disease, and arteriosclerosis are inseparably associated; in the future, the exact role of B₆ in their prevention must be pinpointed.

I would strongly suggest that research be undertaken on the relationship between heart disease and the elasticity of the blood vessels as it was discussed in Chapter 10. This could lead to a lowering of death rate from heart disease in this country. The steroid association with diabetes and heart disease is strong, and B₆ is probably an intermediary that could be preventive in heart disease.

I have taken great pains to emphasize that I am not claiming that B₆ relieves diabetes or prevents heart disease. But the vitamin is helpful to a patient with either of these diseases, and it *may* well be a factor in their prevention. One diabetic patient, for instance, was taking thirty units of insulin at the beginning of B₆ therapy; five years later the patient was still taking thirty units of insulin. There had been no deterioration, but neither had there been any respite from the insulin dose. As seen in Chapter 10, the two men whose EKGs are shown both had myocardial infarctions. They also failed the QEW test. Whether B₆ might have prevented those two coronaries if they had started taking it much, much earlier, perhaps in their childhood, cannot be stated with certainty. What is certain, however, is that all these patients, suffering from diabetes and heart disease, did need B_6 for relief of related signs and symptoms.

One of the most dramatic proofs of B_6's aid is seen in the blind diabetic. Quite often the blind diabetic loses the sense of touch in his fingers. He cannot then read Braille, his last link with the visual world. But B_6 remedies this, restoring his sense of touch and enabling him again to read Braille. It would be difficult to evaluate how much this is worth to the blind diabetic.

Other beneficial effects of B_6 might even be said to hold certain economic significance. The diabetic seamstress, N. H., discussed in Chapter 9, was on government subsidies, or welfare, because she couldn't work. But after B_6 had solved her medical problems in the hands, she was able to make her living *completely* by working at her sewing. Might not others similarly benefit? How many other persons in this nation would like to be well enough to work again, to use their hands, and get off welfare? The answer is likely to be a high figure.

There are millions of persons who would benefit in ways that would prove to be dramatic.

Government, as well as several sectors of our economy, must be involved. The U. S. Department of Agriculture inspects meat and milk all the time. It should also continually monitor what people are buying and provide trained nutritionists in the big chain stores for consultation with the consumers. The government should also establish monitoring stations manned by technicians trained in assessing B_6 deficiency, among others, if we are going to make a serious effort to relieve malnutrition in this country.

In order to preserve a proper mineral balance in our national dietary, the USDA and the Food and Drug Administration should monitor our food supplies and establish standards for the mineral content of vegetables, for instance, whether they are sold in health-food stores or in grocery stores. Biochemists now face the additional challenge of finding new and simple methods of determining B_6 deficiency among the population.

Agriculture will hold a key to our future battle for proper nutrition. The old merry-go-round of what kind of fertilizer is best is not going to be answered except in one way: chemical analysis of the products that go to the marketplace for the consumers. Soils in different parts of the country are different; temperatures and rainfall are different; agricultural practices are different. The best solution for consumers, without question, is to establish standards of what constitutes marketable produce—vegetables and fruit, in particular—with vitamin and mineral content taken into account, and then *establish plant-testing laboratories manned by the best of scientists to determine if the standards are being maintained for the consumers.* As seen in Chapter 11, all that is lush and green is not balanced in nutrients. The study of grass tetany, reported in that chapter, told very clearly that looks can be most deceiving; the grass looked green, lush, and nourishing, everything one would expect from grass, but it caused grass tetany that imperiled the lives of the cattle feeding on it because it was causing low serum magnesium. The soils of this country, and the nutrients in them, are different. Although many standards have been established already, standards for nutrients in food are not among these.

Government cannot do everything for us. We, whether one is a member of the medical profession or the "man in the street," must do our share, too. Dentists, for example, should be taught and trained to the point that they would be among the very best nutritionists, for they are often the first to see clinical evidence of malnutrition, in the gums, teeth, and tongues of patients afflicted with improper eating habits. The dental profession has always been closely allied with the medical profession in this field; dentists must be called on, increasingly in the future, to accept this most valuable role. Dentists can be readily educated in the needed chemistry and nutrition, but as one dentist friend of mine has pointed out, "The medical profession will have to lead in the education and liaison between the two professions in controlling malnutrition."

But education itself should begin at home. We must learn to protect ourselves by eating properly. Every housewife must, in a sense, become a nutritionist, and the impetus for the child should continue into kindergarten and then continue through all school.

Every school child should learn arithmetic by totalling milligrams of pyridoxine and milliequivalents of potassium or magnesium. Why not make calories and nutritional substances a basis for calculations, both mathematical and chemical? Nutrition should be taught by the most able teachers in a school system. Nutrition should be the major course of study in the universities for those teachers who will be teaching health and physical education in grade and high schools.

Government backing, of course, will be essential all up and down the line. The Bureau of Standards could help by insisting not only on clean food but also well-labeled food that would include cautions about preparation and preservation of vitamins and minerals. Here, legislation might be helpful. There is too much at stake and too many people involved; we must make the strongest effort we can.

The scientist, most of all, must not be overlooked. His contributions have been essential to what we now know; they will be just as vital in the future. It has been said that it is the gentle wind that changes things. The patient, gentle approach of many scientists in laboratories around the world has prepared the way for these discoveries relating to B_6. They continue to put together the many answers we are still seeking in regard to B_6.

When I attended the New York Academy of Sciences conference in 1969 I learned that some of the best scientists are quiet, unobtrusive persons who tend to shun arguments or controversy. Many non-scientists don't realize this. This fact itself puts many scientists at a disadvantage when explaining their findings or positions publicly. Certainly they are in no position to go before Congressional committees and do battle with superbly trained lawyers representing large segments of the food industry. On more than one occasion, some of our best scientists have walked out of committee hearings because their positions were presented—unfairly—as being untenable.

There have been unpleasant moments when distinguished scientists have become the targets of glibly uttered half-truths until they sometimes were baited to the point of absurdity. Any seeming weakness is then again pounced on subsequently by those with the half-truth. For this reason, the patient-consumer must learn more about what the truth is in nutrition, and he will have to learn how to exert sufficient political influence in Washington at least to preserve the opportunity to purchase his own supplements.

In today's complex world one finds learning the details of proper nutrition to be quite complicated. The old idea of saying, "Yes, a fellow can get all he needs from food," and eating whatever one wants, has to be discarded. Too few persons know that much about which foods to eat, which nutrients are needed, although the number of the knowledgeable is growing. The real answer is to provide supernutrition, as Dr. Roger Williams has proposed. The people of this country should have supernutrition available so that they can obtain it inexpensively.

The average patient-consumer may be confused about many of the details of proper nutrition, especially when scientists themselves differ. For this reason the consumer-patient is entitled to have the pertinent information explained to him in a way he can understand. This sometimes is a painstaking chore. In all of my writings and lectures I have never once criticized my medical colleagues on this or any other score. Most doctors find each day full of work and responsibilities and they suffer their own anxieties over desperately ill patients. But doctors and other scientists must give more time to the patient-consumer to explain nutritional concepts. It takes time, a lot of time—even weeks and months. When a person has never had a single lecture in chemistry he cannot be expected to master the proper concepts of nutrition in the span of a few minutes.

When a physician treats an ignorant man he has to do the best he can without losing patience with one who has not had the opportunity of extensive academic training. Thousands—perhaps millions—of persons are sincerely interested in food and nutrition today; they take time from their vacations, paying out their hard-earned money, to receive a few crumbs of information from the thin line of professionals who will get down on a speaking level to converse with them. Each year the audiences, all over the nation, have grown. They come to lectures, hungering for nutritional knowledge, sacrificing their time and money to attend. This concept of educating all of our patients-consumers must spread and its need be recognized by all our doctors and other scientists.

The patient and the doctor are both involved in the pursuit of a common goal: health. For this reason, a well-informed patient is as desirable as a competent doctor. As the patient becomes better informed, the physician is served notice to be aware of all discoveries that may promote the health and welfare of the patient. This is as it should be. No man or profession has, or should have, exclusive ownership of medical knowledge. It is for all.

These truth-hungering patients-consumers often pay taxes to support the university professionals who, many times, won't bother to answer letters about nutrition, much less give a lecture to some interested group. This causes mistrust on the part of the patient-consumer and even plays its part in impeding financial assistance for research, farther down the line. Non-scientists need to know more about nutrition; often these are the persons, in research, who can illuminate them.

There are many scientists, now retired as emeritus professors, who could be enlisted in this great national crusade and who would enjoy being a significant part of such a nationwide educational program. Organizations such as the American Cancer Society and the American Heart Association have been quite successful in a number of ways. Perhaps we also need an American Nutrition Society, organized with state and local chapters that would have as a common goal the prevention of malnutrition in America. Dedicated, well-trained nutritionists should lead these programs, with help from both clinical and university scientists.

The state of the union is intimately linked to the state of our nutrition. Without a healthy people we cannot continue to be a vigorous nation. The impetus for moving toward a better, healthful national dietary—which would include sufficient B_6 as well as other essential nutrients—must come from many directions, from many levels of life. It must begin with the earliest time in the individual and proceed through his declining years. As Roger Williams has proclaimed, supernutrition must begin with the fetus, and it must be maintained from infancy on, if we are to prevent later crippling and deadly disease.

And it must include a bountiful supply of vitamin B_6.

Appendix: Additional
Case Histories

Two cases briefly presented in Chapter 7, "B$_6$ During Pregnancy," are described in more detail in this appendix.

CASE 1

S. S., twenty, first pregnancy, a severe diabetic, had developed diabetes in 1968 and had taken the drug tolbutamide until February 1970, when it was replaced by twenty to thirty units of insulin daily. For about three years she had been taking a multivitamin capsule containing 50 milligrams of pyridoxine.

At her first office visit on March 4, 1970, when she was about four months pregnant, she was given a prenatal capsule and pyridoxine that insured her 125 milligrams daily. The capsule also contained 100 milligrams of magnesium oxide and 1 milligram of magnesium sulfate.

A few weeks later edema of the hands had become progressively more apparent. By July 7 her wedding rings had to be removed, and elastic stockings were used to control the edema in her feet and ankles. Although pyridoxine was increased to 425 milligrams daily, it had little effect on the edema.

At 9:00 P.M. on July 30 the patient developed lower abdominal cramping pains, and at 2:15 A.M. that night she was admitted to the hospital in active labor. At the time her blood pressure was 144/100, and she had 4-plus albuminuria. At 7:00 A.M. her blood sugar was 77 milligrams percent and blood pressure was 160/100.

An injection of 100 milligrams of pyridoxine was given at 8:10 A.M., *but no insulin was given.*

An X-ray examination confirmed that the fetus was large, and it was in a breech position. Having decided that a Caesarean section would reduce the hazard for the fetus, I began operating at 9:48 A.M. and soon afterward delivered a ten-pound, seven-and-one-half-ounce male infant that appeared normal and cried spontaneously. Two c.c. of oxytocin was injected into the uterus, and the necessary closures were performed.

While on the operating table the patient received 500 c.c. of lactated Ringer's solution intravenously while preparation was made to receive a pint of blood. Following the blood she received in the recovery room 500 c.c. of normal saline. *It is important to note that these solutions did not contain magnesium.*

By 11:00 A.M. the patient S. S. was awake and talking to the recovery-room nurse. At that time she was injected with 100 milligrams of pyridoxine and all seemed to be well. At 11:30 A.M., however, she complained of something happening to her left arm, and she promptly developed a *grand mal* convulsion. As soon as it could be done, at 11:40 A.M., she was given three grains of sodium phenobarbital and three grains of sodium dilantin by injection. Again at 12:10 P.M. she was injected with one and one half grains of sodium phenobarbital and one and one half grains of sodium dilantin.

Shortly before 1:10 P.M. she had another *grand mal* convulsive seizure, at which time her blood pressure was 200/120 and her blood sugar was 178 milligrams percent, far above normal. At 2:10 P.M. she was awake, with eyes open, talking coherently, and apparently doing well. At 2:45 P.M. her blood pressure was 120/98, and 200 milligrams of pyridoxine were given intravenously. At 3:30 P.M., because she complained of a lower abdominal pain, I gave her 75 milligrams of meperidine, a pain killer, by injection. At 5:20 P.M. she was again given 200 milligrams of pyridoxine intravenously and one and one half grains of sodium phenobarbital.

At no time during the afternoon was the patient sound asleep. From time to time she talked with relatives. Blood sugar at 4:00 P.M. had leaped to 236 milligrams percent. At 5:30 P.M. she was given ten units of regular insulin by hypodermic injection, and at 6:00 P.M. she went into violent *grand mal* convulsions that continued until magnesium sulfate (1,250 milligrams) was given intravenously at 8:10 P.M., when convulsions ceased and the patient went to sleep. About the same time, 1,000 milligrams of magnesium sulfate were also given by intramuscular injection. Approximately an hour earlier she had been given 10 milligrams of reserpine by intramuscular injection, to no avail.

The patient had no more convulsions after the injection of magnesium sulfate, and at 9:05 P.M. she was resting quietly with a blood pressure of 145/80. Magnesium sulfate and reserpine were given by injection at eight-hour intervals for the next twenty-four hours. The reserpine was given only because a consulting colleague suggested it, but it is doubtful that it had anything to do with relief from the convulsions. Both mother and child survived the great ordeal, and, after July 31, which was the day of parturition, both did quite well. On August 4 a catheterized urine specimen was negative for red blood cells, casts, and albumin, and on August 5 mother and child were discharged from the hospital, both in good condition.

CASE 2

V. M., twenty-four, was pregnant for the first time. She was first examined on June 15, 1971, then about two months pregnant. Blood pressure was normal at 130/80, and urine was negative for albumin, casts, and red blood cells.

Her family history was of some interest because her paternal grandfather had died in 1946 while undergoing amputation of an extremity involved in diabetic gangrene. One of her paternal grand-aunts was also a diabetic and was known to require insulin.

The patient V. M. worked in a chicken-processing plant where she stood beside a conveyor belt and grasped about 5,000 chickens a day with her left hand and opened the chickens with a large pair of scissors with her right hand. Thus her hands were exercised constantly each day on her job.

At the time of her first office visit I prescribed 50 milligrams of pyridoxine morning and night along with a multivitamin-mineral capsule that also contained 25 milligrams of pyridoxine. This gave her a total of 125 milligrams of pyridoxine daily.

Her pregnancy proceeded smoothly until August 8, when she developed pain and swelling in her left hand. A few days later, on August 11, she did not report to work because of the increased swelling and loss of sensation in her left thumb, index, and long fingers. But on August 12 and 13 she returned to work in spite of the swelling and disturbed sensation.

On August 14 she reported to my office for a physical examination, and I found her to have painful flexion of the interphalangeal joints of the left hand but not of the right hand on which there was a callus from her work. She complained of "numbness, tingling, and a dead sensation" in the thumb, index, and long fingers of the left hand when I lightly tapped at the carpal tunnel, in the wrist. Other aspects were normal; urine was negative for sugar and albumin and her blood pressure remained at 130/80.

I instructed her to take a total of 325 milligrams of pyridoxine daily and to try to remain on the job and at work.

When I next saw her at 4:00 P.M. on August 17, three days after increasing the dosage of pyridoxine, she had perfect flexion of all fingers of her left hand. There was some slight residual subjective stiffness as compared with the right hand, but objectively all swelling had subsided and the left hand seemed normal.

"My left hand doesn't hurt or pain like it did three days ago," she said. "My fingers feel numb at the tips"—she pointed to the thumb, index, and long fingers—"but my hand does not hurt like it did."

My tapping the left carpal tunnel caused tingling in the long finger but none in the thumb or index finger.

That day and the day before she had handled, as usual, about 5,000 chickens, working until 3:00 P.M. each day.

She was to continue taking 325 milligrams of pyridoxine daily.

On September 11, when she was seen next, she had no swelling in the hands or feet, but she said she had a barely perceptible numbness in the tips of the thumb, index, and long fingers of her left hand. By then she was five months pregnant, and during the previous four days she had opened her usual 5,000 chickens each day. Urine was negative for sugar and albumin, and blood pressure was steady at 130/80. She had not been absent from work since I had increased the pyridoxine to 325 milligrams daily.

She said she was planning to discontinue work—for no particular reason except for her general comfort and because she wanted to get more rest. I reduced the B_6 dosage to 125 milligrams daily, since she had no edema or discomfort in her hands.

On December 21, in her ninth month of pregnancy, she had edema of the feet but said there was no numbness or tingling in her hands. However, her blood pressure had shot up to 180/120, and there was albumin in her urine, recorded as 1-plus. On the positive side, there were no sugar, casts, or red blood cells in the urine. A diagnosis of toxemia was made.

From previous clinical experience it seemed certain that the third condition of eclampsia could be prevented. Accordingly I instructed her to resume taking 325 milligrams of pyridoxine daily, and in addition to the B_6 and the multivitamin-mineral capsule she had been taking since her first office visit, I added magnesium and potassium. The daily dosage of 325 milligrams of pyridoxine was divided into three doses and was now given with magnesium aspartate (500 milligrams morning and night) and potassium aspartate (500 milligrams morning and night). Thus she was also receiving daily 1,000 milligrams of magnesium and 1,000 milligrams of potassium.

During the next two weeks there was a reduction of the edema in her hands and feet.

At 1:00 A.M. on January 13, 1972—*twenty-two days after initiating the additional therapy with magnesium and potassium*—V. M. began painful uterine contractions and was in labor. She was admitted to the hospital at 12:40 P.M. that same day with an extremely high blood pressure of 210/110 and albuminuria designated as 2-plus (100 milligrams percent). The cervix was dilated three centimeters.

There was absolutely no edema in her hands or feet. One could see the outline of every tendon on the back of her hands and the top of her feet.

The drama of her hospital stay was recorded in this sequence:

12:40 P.M.—200 milligrams of pyridoxine given by injection.

5:45 P.M.—Cervix dilated five centimeters. Patient given one-fourth grain of morphine sulfate and 1/200 grain of scopolamine by injection.

6:05 P.M.—500 milligrams of magnesium aspartate and 500 milligrams of potassium aspartate given by mouth.

6:15 P.M.—Amniotic membranes ruptured.

8:30 P.M.—200 milligrams of pyridoxine injected. Fasting blood sugar level at 108 milligrams percent.

10:44 P.M.—Without episiotomy or forceps and without laceration, a seven-pound, two-and-one-half-ounce female infant was delivered, crying spontaneously and appearing normal. A catheterized urine specimen taken on the delivery table revealed a 2-plus albuminuria (100 milligrams percent) with no casts or red blood cells in the urine. During a very strenuous hour and a half on the delivery table she experienced no leg cramps and suffered no headache. Her blood pressure ranged from 200/90 to 210/110 while on the delivery table.

11:15 P.M.—500 milligrams of magnesium aspartate and 500 milligrams of potassium asparate given by mouth.

January 14, 7:00 A.M.—100 milligrams of pyridoxine given by injection.

5:30 P.M. (the day after birth)—Blood pressure 170/100.

January 15, 10:00 A.M.—Blood pressure 168/90. Catheterized urine specimen showed no red blood cells and two to three white blood cells. (The day of discharge, less than thirty-six hours after giving birth.)

On discharge on January 15 the infant was taking a formula well and seemed normal.

In summary, V. M., the mother patient, was never given a diuretic or an antihypertensive drug even though her blood pressure twenty-two days before parturition had reached 180/120 and there was objective edema in the hands and feet, and she had albuminuria. All trace of edema disappeared when pyridoxine was increased and magnesium and potassium added. Her blood pressure of 210/110, not existing as such before pregnancy, and the 2-plus albuminuria constituted a diagnosis of toxemia of pregnancy. During twenty-one hours and forty-four minutes of labor, the very courageous patient was given only one sedative, a single injection of morphine and scopolamine. The patient, suffering from toxemia, including hypertension and albuminuria, did not have edema on admission to the hospital, and she did not convulse. I wish to emphasize that oxytocin and ergonovine were withheld following parturition. *It also cannot be overemphasized that during the prenatal period V. M. had all the signs and symptoms of the carpal tunnel syndrome associated with pregnancy—which responded to an increased dosage of pyridoxine within three days and without taking time off from her strenuous job.*

Source Notes

PREFACE

1. Snell, E. E., Guirard, B. M., and Williams, R. S., "Occurrence in Natural Products of a Physiologically Active Metabolite of Pyridoxine," *Journal of Biological Chemistry* 143, pp. 519–30, 1942.

2. Braunstein, A. E., "Pyridoxal phosphate," in: *The Enzymes,* edited by P. D. Boyer, H. A. Lardy and K. Myrbäck. New York: Academic Press, Vol. 2, pp. 113–84, 1960.

3. Sauberlich, H. E., in *The Vitamins,* edited by W. H. Sebrell, Jr., and R. S. Harris, Vol. 2, p. 44 ff., 1968.

2. THE SLEEPING GIANT OF NUTRITION

1. *Webster's New World Dictionary of the American Language, College Edition* (Cleveland and New York: The World Publishing Co., 1966), p. 1185.

2. In tracing the history of vitamin B_6 from this point to its chemical isolation in 1938 the authors will be drawing primarily on, as a guide and reference, Dr. György's concise but thorough "Developments Leading to the Metabolic Role of Vitamin B_6," *American Journal of Clinical Nutrition* (October 1971), Vol. 24, pp. 1250–56.

3. György, Paul, "The History of Vitamin B_6. Introductory Remarks," *Vitamins and Hormones* (1964), Vol. 22, pp. 361–65.

234   SOURCE NOTES

4. Spies, Tom D., Bean, William B., and Ashe, William F., "A Note on the Use of Vitamin B_6 in Human Nutrition," *Journal of the American Medical Association* (June 10, 1939), pp. 2414–15. See also "24-Hour Recoveries Result from Synthesized Vitamin," *Science News Letter* (June 24, 1939), p. 395.

5. *Science News Letter* (June 1, 1940), p. 340.

6. Lepkovsky, Samuel, Roboz, Elisabeth, and Haagen-Smit, A. J., "Xanthurenic Acid and Its Role in the Tryptophan Metabolism of Pyridoxine-Deficient Rats," *Journal of Biological Chemistry* (1943), Vol. 149, pp. 195–201.

7. For a discussion of this, see Wachstein, Max, "Evidence for a Relative Vitamin B_6 Deficiency in Pregnancy and Some Disease States," *Vitamins and Hormones* (1964), Vol. 22, pp. 705–19.

8. György, "Developments Leading to Metabolic Role of B_6."

9. General readers will find a report on this episode by Howard Glassford in *Today's Health* (December 1954), pp. 26–27, 44. Also see *Vitamin B_6 in Human Nutrition: Report of the Tenth M & R Pediatric Research Conference* (Columbus, Ohio, M & R Laboratories, 1954, 59 pp.).

10. See Vilter, Richard W., "The Vitamin B_6-Hydrazide Relationship," *Vitamins and Hormones* (1964), Vol. 22, pp. 797–805.

11. A review of B_6 in relation to anemia can be found in Harris, John W., and Horrigan, Daniel L., "Pyridoxine-Responsive Anemia— Prototype and Variations on the Theme," *Vitamins and Hormones* (1964), Vol. 22, pp. 721–53.

12. György, "Developments." Walter B. Cannon, M.D. (1871–1945), was an American physiologist.

13. S. V., "Serendipitous Sulphonylureas," *Journal of the American Medical Association* (March 6, 1972), Vol. 219, No. 10, p. 1335.

14. Morrison, L. M., "Diet in Coronary Atherosclerosis," *Journal of the American Medical Association* (June 25, 1960), Vol. 173, pp. 884–88.

15. One result of my clinical experience in these years was a plea for more protein rather than fat in beef production, made at the Western Hemisphere Nutrition Congress in Chicago in November 1965. See Ellis, John M., "Addendum A: Development of Food Products," *Proceedings, Western Hemisphere Nutrition Congress* (Chicago: American Medical Association, 1966), pp. 247–48.

16. Ellis, John M., *The Doctor Who Looked at Hands* (New York: Vantage Press, 1966), pp. 147–150.

3. RHEUMATISM—AS OLD AS THE GREEKS

1. Bender, George A., and Thom, Robert A., *A History of Medicine in Pictures* (Parke, Davis & Co., 1958), Vol. 2, unpaged.

2. Spiera, H., "Excretion of Tryptophan Metabolites in Rheumatoid Arthritis," *Arthritis and Rheumatism* (April 1966), Vol. 9, No. 2, pp. 318–24.

3. Bett, Isobel M., "Urinary Tryptophan Metabolites in Rheumatoid Arthritis and Some Other Diseases," *Annals of the Rheumatic Diseases* (1966), Vol. 25, pp. 556–62.

4. Bett, Isobel M., "Effect of Pyridoxine on Tryptophan Metabolism in Rheumatoid Arthritis," *Annals of the Rheumatic Diseases* (1962), Vol. 21, p. 388.

5. McKusick, Anne B., and Hsu, Jeng M., "Clinical and Metabolic Studies of the Shoulder-Hand Syndrome in Tuberculosis Patients," *Arthritis and Rheumatism* (1961), Vol. 4, p. 426.

4. RHEUMATISM AND THE CARPAL TUNNEL SYNDROME

1. Phalen, G. S., "Reflections on 21 Years' Experience With the Carpal-Tunnel Syndrome," *Journal of the American Medical Association* (1970), Vol. 212, No. 8, pp. 1365–67.

2. Jones, Ernest, *The Life and Work of Sigmund Freud* (New York: Basic Books, 1953–1955; 2 vols.), especially Vol. 2, pp. 28, 82.

3. For the Putnam–Freud correspondence, see *James Jackson Putnam and Psychoanalysis: Letters Between Putnam and Sigmund Freud, Ernest Jones, William James, Sandor Ferenczi, and Morton Prince, 1877–1917* (Cambridge, Mass.: Harvard University Press, 1971), ed. Nathan G. Hale, Jr. Trans. Judith Bernays Heller.

4. Phalen, *op. cit.*

5. Taylor, Neal, "Special Review: Carpal Tunnel Syndrome," *American Journal of Physical Medicine* (August 1971), Vol. 50, No. 4, pp. 192–213.

6. Cannon, B. W., and Love, J. G., "Tardy Median Palsy; Median Neuritis; Median Thenar Neuritis Amenable to Surgery," *Surgery* (1946), Vol. 20, pp. 210–16.

7. Brain, W. R., Wright, A. D., and Wilkinson, M., "Spontaneous Compression of Both Median Nerves in Carpal Tunnel," *Lancet* (1947), No. 1, pp. 277–82.

8. Phalen, *op. cit.*

9. Ellis, John M., *The Doctor Who Looked at Hands* (New York: Vantage Press, 1966).

10. Ellis, John M., "Vitamin B_6 in Treatment of the Carpal Tunnel and Shoulder-Hand Syndromes," *Journal of Applied Nutrition* (Winter 1972), Vol. 24, Nos. 3–4, pp. 73 ff.

11. Sabour, M. S., and Fadel, H. E., "The Carpal-Tunnel Syndrome —A New Complication Ascribed to the 'Pill,' " *American Journal of Obstetrics and Gynecology* (1970), Vol. 107, No. 8, pp. 1265–66.

12. Tobin, S. M., "Carpal Tunnel Syndrome in Pregnancy," *American Journal of Obstetrics and Gynecology* (1967), Vol. 97, No. 4, pp. 493–98.

13. Wachstein, M., and Gudaitis, A., "Disturbance of Vitamin B_6 Metabolism in Pregnancy," *Journal of Laboratory and Clinical Medicine* (October 1952), Vol. 40, pp. 550–57.

14. Rose, D. P., "Excretion of Xanthurenic Acid in the Urine of Women Taking Progestrogen-Oestrogen Preparations," *Nature* (1966), Vol. 210, pp. 196–97.

15. Phillips, R. S., "Carpal Tunnel Syndrome as a Manifestation of Systemic Disease," *Annals of the Rheumatic Diseases* (1967), Vol. 26, p. 59.

6. THE BIRTH-CONTROL PILL

1. Ellis, John M., *The Doctor Who Looked at Hands* (New York: Vantage Press, 1966), p. 298.

2. Rose, D. P., "Excretion of Xanthurenic Acid in the Urine of Women Taking Progestrogen-Oestrogen Preparations," *Nature* (1966), Vol. 210, pp. 196–97.

3. Baumblatt, Michael J., and Winston, Frank, "Pyridoxine and the Pill," *Lancet* (April 18, 1970), No. 1, pp. 832–33.

7. B_6 DURING PREGNANCY

1. Klieger, Jack A., Altshuler, Charles H., Krakow, G., and Hollister, C., "Abnormal Pyridoxine Metabolism in Toxemia of Pregnancy," *Vitamin B_6 in Metabolism of the Nervous System (Annals of the New York Academy of Sciences*, Vol. 166, Art. 1, Sept. 30, 1960), pp. 288–96.

8. LIFE BEFORE, AND AFTER, BIRTH

1. Bunnell, R. H., "Meetings: Vitamin B_6," *Science* (October 30, 1964), Vol. 146, pp. 674–77.

2. Krebs, Edwin G., and Fischer, Edmond H., "Phosphorylase and Related Enzymes of Glycogen Metabolism," *Vitamins and Hormones* (1964), Vol. 22, pp. 399–410.

3. Hunt, Andrew D., Jr., Stokes, Joseph, Jr., McCrory, Wallace W., and Stroud, H. H., "Pyridoxine Dependency: Report of a Case of Intractable Convulsions in an Infant Controlled by Pyridoxine," *Pediatrics* (1954), Vol. 13, pp. 140–45.

4. For an excellent, authoritative examination and review of this subject, see David Baird Coursin, "Vitamin B$_6$ Metabolism in Infants and Children," *Vitamins and Hormones* (1964), Vol. 22, pp. 755–86.

5. György, Paul, "Concluding Remarks," *Vitamins and Hormones* (1964), Vol. 22, p. 885.

6. Ellis, John M., *The Doctor Who Looked at Hands* (New York: Vantage Press, 1966), pp. 237–39.

9. THE MYSTERY OF DIABETES

1. The tryptophan–niacin pathway is diagrammed on p. 1252 in Paul György's "Developments Leading to the Metabolic Role of Vitamin B$_6$," *The American Journal of Clinical Nutrition* (October 1971), Vol. 24, pp. 1250–56.

2. Wacker, Warren E. C., and Parisi, Alfred F., "Magnesium Metabolism," *New England Journal of Medicine* (March 21, 28, April 4, 1968), Vol. 278, pp. 658–63, 712–27, 772–76.

3. Jackson, Charles E., and Meier, Donald W., "Routine Serum Magnesium Analysis: Correlation With Clinical State in 5,100 Patients," *Annals of Internal Medicine* (October 1968), Vol. 69, No. 4, pp. 743–48.

4. Somjen, G., Hilmy, M., and Stephen, C. R., "Failure to Anesthetize Human Subjects by Intravenous Administration of Magnesium Sulfate," *The Journal of Pharmacology and Experimental Therapeutics* (1966), Vol. 154, No. 2, pp. 652–59.

10. HEART DISEASE AND B$_6$

1. Ellis, John M., *The Doctor Who Looked at Hands* (New York: Vantage Press, 1966), pp. 174–76.

2. *Turning-Points in Cardiovascular Medicine, I:* reprint of "Pectoris Dolor" from William Heberden's *Commentaries on the History and Cure of Diseases,* published in facsimile by Merck Sharp & Dohme, West Point, Pennsylvania.

3. Grollman, Arthur, *Essentials of Endocrinology* (Philadelphia, London, Montreal: J. B. Lippincott, Co., 1947; 2nd ed.), p. 473.

11. WHEN LABORATORY AND CLINIC AGREE

1. For a major technical contribution on this subject, see Snell, Esmond E., and Haskell, Betty E., "The Metabolism of Vitamin B₆," in *Comprehensive Biochemistry,* ed. Marcel Florkin and Elmer R. Stotz (New York, Elsevier Publishing Co., 1971), Vol. 21, pp. 47–71.

2. Borsook, Henry, "The Relation of the Vitamin B₆ Human Requirement to the Amount in the Diet," *Vitamins and Hormones* (1964), Vol. 22, pp. 855–74.

3. Sauberlich, Howerde E., "IX. Biochemical Systems and Biochemical Detection of Deficiency," *The Vitamins: Chemistry, Physiology, Pathology, Methods,* ed. W. H. Sebrell, Jr., and Robert S. Harris (New York and London: Academic Press, 1968; 2nd ed.) Vol. II, pp. 44–80.

4. Sebrell, W. H. Jr., "The Importance of Vitamin B₆ in Human Nutrition," *Vitamins and Hormones* (1964), Vol. 22, pp. 875–84.

5. Fuller, Henry L., "Vitamin B₆ in Farm Animal Nutrition and Pets," *ibid.,* pp. 659–76.

6. Williams, Mary Ann, "Vitamin B₆ and Amino Acids—Recent Research in Animals," *ibid.,* pp. 561–79.

7. Canham, J. E., Baker, E. M., Harding, R. S., Sauberlich, H. E., and Plough, I. C., "Dietary Protein—Its Relationship to Vitamin B₆ Requirements and Function," *Vitamin B₆ in Metabolism of the Nervous System (Annals of the New York Academy of Sciences;* September 30, 1969, Vol. 166, Art. 1), pp. 16–29. See also Sauberlich, H. E., "Human Requirements for Vitamin B₆," *Vitamins and Hormones* (1964), Vol. 22, pp. 807–23.

8. Sebrell, *op. cit.*

9. Mason, Merle, Ford, Jonathan, and Wu, Helen L. C., "Effects of Steroid and Nonsteroid Metabolites on Enzyme Conformation and Pyridoxal Phosphate Binding," *Vitamin B₆ in Metabolism of the Nervous System,* pp. 170–83.

10. Rose, David P., "Excretion of Xanthurenic Acid in the Urine of Women Taking Progestogen-Oestrogen Preparations," *Nature* (April 9, 1966), Vol. 210, pp. 196–97.

11. Price, J. M., Thornton, Madeline J., and Mueller, Lois M., "Tryptophan Metabolism in Women Using Steroid Hormones for Ovulation Control," *The American Journal of Clinical Nutrition* (May 1967), Vol. 20, No. 5, pp. 452–56.

12. Toseland, P. A., and Price, Sarah, "Tryptophan and Oral Contraceptives," *British Medical Journal* (March 22, 1969), No. 5646, p. 777.

13. Brown, R. R., Rose, D. P., Price, J. M., and Wolf, H., "Tryptophan Metabolism as Affected by Anovulatory Agents," *Vitamin B₆ in Metabolism of the Nervous System,* pp. 44–56.

14. Luhby, A. Leonard, Brin, Myron, Gordon, Myron, Davis, Patricia, Murphy, Maureen, and Spiegel, Herbert, "Vitamin B₆ Metabolism in Users of Oral Contraceptive Agents. I. Abnormal Urinary Xanthurenic Acid Excretion and Its Correction by Pyridoxine," *The American Journal of Clinical Nutrition* (June 1971), Vol. 24, No. 6, pp. 684–93.

15. Sprince, Herbert, Lowy, Richard S., Folsome, Clair E., and Behrman, Johannes S., "Studies on the Urinary Excretion of 'Xanthurenic Acid' During Normal and Abnormal Pregnancy: A Survey of the Excretion of 'Xanthurenic Acid' in Normal Non-pregnant, Normal Pregnant, Pre-Eclamptic, and Eclamptic Women," *The American Journal of Obstetrics and Gynecology* (July 1951), Vol. 62, pp. 84–92.

16. Wachstein, M., and Gudaitis, A., "Disturbance of Vitamin B₆ Metabolism in Pregnancy," *Journal of Laboratory and Clinical Medicine* (1952), Vol. 40, pp. 550–57.

17. Wachstein, Max, "Evidence for a Relative Vitamin B₆ Deficiency in Pregnancy and Some Disease States," *Vitamins and Hormones* (1964), Vol. 22, pp. 705–19.

18. Tobin, Sidney M., "Carpal Tunnel Syndrome in Pregnancy," *American Journal of Obstetrics and Gynecology* (February 15, 1967), Vol. 97, pp. 493–98.

19. Klieger, Jack A., Altshuler, Charles H., Krakow, G., and Hollister, C., "Abnormal Pyridoxine Metabolism in Toxemia of Pregnancy," *Vitamin B₆ in Metabolism of the Nervous System*, pp. 288–96.

20. Coursin, David Baird, "Vitamin B₆ Metabolism in Infants and Children," *Vitamins and Hormones* (1964), Vol. 22, pp. 755–86.

21. Coursin, David B., "Vitamin B₆ and Brain Function in Animals and Man," *Vitamin B₆ in Metabolism of the Nervous System* (1969), pp. 7–15.

22. Hansson, Olle, "Tryptophan Loading and Pyridoxine Treatment in Children with Epilepsy," *ibid.*, pp. 306–09.

23. Raine, D. N., "Effect of Treatment on Tryptophan Metabolism in Childhood Epilepsy," *ibid.*, pp. 297–305.

24. Davis, Starkey D., Nelson, Thomas, and Shepard, Thomas H.,

"Teratogenicity of Vitamin B_6 Deficiency: Omphalocele, Skeletal and Neural Defects, and Splenic Hypoplasia," *Science* (September 25, 1970), Vol. 169, pp. 1329–30.

25. Wiss, Oswald, and Weber, Fritz, "Biochemical Pathology of Vitamin B_6 Deficiency," *Vitamins and Hormones* (1964), Vol. 22, pp. 495–501.

26. Axelrod, A. E., and Trakatellis, Anthony C., "Relationship of Pyridoxine to Immunological Phenomena," *ibid.*, pp. 591–607.

27. Hale, Fred, "Pigs Born Without Eye Balls," *Journal of Heredity* (March 1933), Vol. XXIV, No. 3, pp. 105–6.

28. Hale, Fred, "The Relation of Vitamin A to the Eye Development in the Pig," *Record of Proceedings, American Society of Animal Production* (Annual Meeting, 1934), pp. 126–28.

29. Hale, Fred, "The Relation of Vitamin A to Anophthalmos in Pigs," *American Journal of Ophthalmology* (December 1935), Vol. 18, No. 12, pp. 1087–92.

30. Hale, Fred, "The Relation of Maternal Vitamin A Deficiency to Microphthalmia in Pigs," *Texas State Journal of Medicine* (July, 1937), Vol. 33, pp. 228–232.

31. White, Abraham, Handler, Philip, Smith, Emil L., and Stetten, DeWitt, Jr., *Principles of Biochemistry* (New York: The Blakiston Division of McGraw-Hill Book Co., Inc., 1959; 2nd ed.), pp. 935–36.

32. Kotake, Yakito, "Experiments of Chronic Diabetic Symptoms Caused by Xanthurenic Acid, an Abnormal Metabolite of Tryptophan," *Clinical Chemistry: Journal of the American Association of Clinical Chemists* (1957), Vol. 3, pp. 432–46.

33. Grodsky, Gerold M., and Bennett, Leslie L., "Effect of Glucose 'Pulse', Glucagon, and the Cations $Ca++$, $Mg++$, and $K+$ on Insulin Secretion *In Vitro*," *Journal of Clinical Investigation* (1966), Vol. 45, p. 1018.

34. Bennett, Leslie L., Curry, Donald L., and Grodsky, Gerold M., "Calcium-Magnesium Antagonism in Insulin Secretion by the Perfused Rat Pancreas," *Endocrinology* (September 1969), Vol. 85, No. 3, pp. 594–96.

35. Whang, R., Wagner, R., Rodgers, D., "The Effect of Intravenous Insulin and Glucose on Serum Mg and K Concentration," *Clinical Research* (1966), Vol. 14, p. 390.

36. Smith, William O., Hammarsten, James F., and Eliel, Leonard P., "The Clinical Expression of Magnesium Deficiency," *Journal of the American Medical Association* (September 3, 1960), Vol. 174, No. 1, pp. 77–78.

37. Maria C. Linder, Ph.D., personal communication.

38. Schroeder, Henry A., Nason, Alexis P., and Tipton, Isabel H., "Essential Metals in Man: Magnesium," *Journal of Chronic Diseases* (April 1969), Vol. 21, No. 11/12, pp. 815–41.

39. Smith, Hammarsen, and Eliel, *op. cit.* For another review of diuretics and magnesium see Wacker, Warren E. C., and Parisi, Alfred F., "Magnesium Metabolism," *New England Journal of Medicine* (March 21, 28; April 4, 1968), Vol. 278, pp. 658–63, 712–27, 772–76.

40. Jackson, Charles E., and Meier, Donald W., "Routine Serum Magnesium Analysis: Correlation with Clinical State in 5,100 Patients," *Annals of Internal Medicine* (October 1968), Vol. 69, No. 4, pp. 743–48.

41. Flowers, C. E., Jr., "Magnesium Sulfate in Obstetrics," *American Journal of Obstetrics and Gynecology* (March 1965), Vol. 91, No. 6, p. 763.

42. E. E. Neal, Jr., personal communication.

43. Wacker and Parisi, *op. cit.*

44. Smith, R. H., "Calcium and Magnesium Metabolism in Calves. 2. Effect of Dietary Vitamin D and Ultraviolet Irradiation of Milk-Fed Calves," *Biochemical Journal* (1958), Vol. 70, pp. 201–5.

45. Greenwald, J. H., Dubin, A., and Cardon, L. C., "Hypo-magnesemic Tetany Due to Excessive Lactation," *American Journal of Medicine* (1963), Vol. 35, pp. 854–60.

46. Mushett, C. W., and Emerson, G., "Arteriosclerosis in Pyridoxine-Deficient Monkeys and Dogs," *Federation Proceedings* (March 1956), Vol. 15, p. 526.

47. Rinehart, James F., and Greenberg, Louis D., "Arteriosclerotic Lesions in Pyridoxine-Deficient Monkeys," *American Journal of Pathology* (1949), Vol. 25, pp. 481–91. Also see Greenberg, Louis D., "Arteriosclerotic, Dental, and Hepatic Lesions in Pyridoxine-Deficient Monkeys," *Vitamins and Hormones* (1964), Vol. 22, pp. 677–94.

48. Gibson, J. B., Carson, Nina A. J., and Neill, D. W., "Pathological Findings in Homocystinuria," *Journal of Clinical Pathology* (July 1964), Vol. 17, No. 4, pp. 427–37.

49. McCully, Kilmer S., "Vascular Pathology of Homocysteinemia: Implications for the Pathogenesis of Arteriosclerosis," *American Journal of Pathology* (July 1969), Vol. 56, No. 1/Whole No. 326, pp. 111–28.

50. McCully, Kilmer S., "Importance of Homocysteine-Induced Abnormalities of Proteoglycan Structure in Arteriosclerosis," *American Journal of Pathology* (April 1970), Vol. 59, No. 1/Whole No. 335, pp. 181–93.

51. McCully, Kilmer S., and Ragsdale, Bruce D., "Production of Arteriosclerosis by Homocysteinemia," *American Journal of Pathology* (October 1970), Vol. 61, No. 1, pp. 1–12.

52. Mueller, John F., "Vitamin B_6 in Fat Metabolism," *Vitamins and Hormones* (1964), Vol. 22, pp. 787–96.

53. Van Woert, Melvin H., "Low Pyridoxine Diet in Parkinsonism," *JAMA* (February 28, 1972), Vol. 219, No. 9, p. 1211.

54. Mars, Harold, Barrera, Elmer Rene, and Bennet, Stephen, "Levodopa and Pyridoxine," *JAMA* (March 27, 1972), Vol. 219, No. 13, p. 1764.

55. Hillman, Robert W., "Effect of Vitamin B_6 on Dental Caries in Man," *Vitamins and Hormones* (1964), Vol. 22, pp. 695–704.

56. Greenberg, Louis D., *op. cit.*

57. Gershoff, Stanley N., "Vitamin B_6 and Oxalate Metabolism," *Vitamins and Hormones* (1964), Vol. 22, pp. 581–89.

12. THE FUTURE: A PROJECTION FOR B_6

1. György, Paul, "Developments Leading to the Metabolic Role of Vitamin B_6," *American Journal of Clinical Nutrition* (October 1971), Vol. 24, pp. 1250–56.

2. Brown, R. R., "Normal and Pathological Conditions Which May Alter the Human Requirement for Vitamin B_6," *Journal of Agriculture and Food Chemistry*.

3. Snell, Esmond E., "Summary of Session I and Some Notes on the Metabolism of Vitamin B_6," *Vitamins and Hormones* (1964), Vol. 22, pp. 485–94 .

4. Borsook, Henry, "The Relation of the Vitamin B_6 Human Requirement to the Amount in the Diet," *ibid.*, pp. 855–74.

5. Hurley, Lucille S., "The Consequences of Fetal Impoverishment," *Nutrition Today* (December 1968), Vol. 3, No. 4, pp. 3–9.

6. Schroeder, Henry A., Nason, Alexis P., and Tipton, Isabel H., "Essential Metals in Man: Magnesium," *Journal of Chronic Diseases* (April 1969), Vol. 21, No. 11/12, pp. 815–41.

Index

About the Authors

DR. JOHN M. ELLIS has been associated with Titus County Memorial Hospital in Mt. Pleasant, Texas, since 1956. At present he is Chief of Medical Staff at Titus. His internship and residencies in pathology and general surgery were spent in St. Louis, Missouri, at the Missouri Pacific Hospital, the Barnard Skin and Cancer Hospital, and the St. Louis City Hospital. Dr. Ellis' clinical research with Vitamin B$_6$ began in 1961, and since then his work done on the subject has received international attention. His first book, *The Doctor Who Looked at Hands*, is an autobiographical account of Dr. Ellis' experiences during the initial phases of his work with the vitamin. Dr. Ellis and his wife, Lucille, have four children. They live in Mt. Pleasant, where, additionally, Dr. Ellis is a prominent breeder of registered Brahman cattle.

JAMES PRESLEY was educated in Texas, where he received his Ph.D. from the University of Texas in 1958. His career in journalism won him a number of top prizes in Texas and Arkansas press association competitions, and he was nominated for the Pulitzer prize in reporting. He is currently a contributing editor to the *Texas Observer*. Mr. Presley has been a free-lance writer since 1962; he specializes in biographical and medical subjects. He has collaborated on two previous books: *Center of the Storm: Memoirs of John T. Scopes* and *"Please, Doctor, Do Something!"* In 1971 he won the Anson Jones Award for excellence in medical writing. Mr. Presley and his wife, Fran, have two children and live in Texarkana, Texas.

73 74 75 76 77 10 9 8 7 6 5 4 3 2 1